THE LEGENDARY QUEST

For Professionals Seeking Inner and Outer Excellence and Authentic Fulfillment

D1713824

DR. KETAN KULKARNI
DR. FRANCIS YOO

Front Cover Image: Painting by Ketan Kulkarni
Independent Published
ISBN: 979-8-4173-2583-0

CONTENTS

Preface -- 1

How to Use This Book ------------------------------------- 5

Introduction -- 7

    Why are Most People Unfulfilled? --------------------- 10

    The Limited-Self Model ------------------------------- 9

PART I: RECOGNIZING THE PROBLEM ------------- 15

Chapter 1: Are You Pursuing Authentic Goals? ----------- 17

    The Irony --- 17

    Success that Becomes No Success -------------------- 19

    Our Measures of Success are Flawed ----------------- 20

    What Do You Really Want? ----------------------------- 21

    We are Submerged in a Matrix ----------------------- 23

    The Dichotomy of Choices ---------------------------- 24

    Look Within Not Without ----------------------------- 26

    Universal Myth: I'll be Happy When... --------------- 28

    References --- 30

Chapter 2: Too Entitled for Your Title -------------------- 33

    What Determines Well-being? ----------------------- 33

    It's Not About the Labels ----------------------------- 34

We Have Got It Wrong and Continue to Do So------ 35

Need of a Comprehensive Framework for Success: Don't Miss the Forest for the Trees ----------------------- 37

Burn-in Not Burn-out ----------------------------- 39

Bring in the Dollars! ----------------------------- 40

What About the Workaholic? -----------------------41

The Double-edged Digital World--------------------- 42

Old Dogs Can't Learn New Tricks... Or Can They? - 43

References -- 45

Chapter 3: Your Core Beliefs are Wrong ------------------ 47

Success is Slow and Hard... Or Is It? ----------------- 47

Long Hours Culture --------------------------------- 49

Missing Out --------------------------------------- 51

The Green Grass ----------------------------------- 53

Sacrificing for the System ------------------------- 54

Cultural Programming ------------------------------ 56

Endless Work-------------------------------------- 57

The Same Dichotomy ------------------------------ 59

References --------------------------------------- 60

PART II: INNER EXCELLENCE ---------------------- 63

Chapter 4: Be Aware ------------------------------- 65

Inside not Outside -------------------------------- 65

The Awareness Model------------------------------ 67

Core Values --- 69

The Core of Your Existence -------------------------- 70

People and Values --------------------------------------- 71

Self-Assessment and Cultivation --------------------- 72

The Power of Now --------------------------------------- 74

Visualizing and Living your Ideal --------------------- 75

Unconscious Direction----------------------------------- 76

Constructive Exercises and Emotional Intelligence -- 78

Managing Emotions ------------------------------------ 80

Influential Thinkers ------------------------------------- 81

Summary--- 83

Further Work and Reading ---------------------------- 84

References --- 84

Chapter 5: Thoughts and Feelings are Optional ---------- 87

Thinking the Thoughts -------------------------------- 87

Responding Emotionally-------------------------------- 89

Taking Ownership -------------------------------------- 90

Negative Self-Talk -------------------------------------- 91

Emotional not Intellectual----------------------------- 93

Tolle's Internal Landscape ----------------------------- 95

Ingroups and Outgroups-------------------------------- 96

Mindfulness Practice------------------------------------ 97

Observing Others --------------------------------------- 98

Physical Place --100

Cultivating Thoughts and Emotions ------------------101

Coaching and Positive Psychology --------------------102

My Titanic Hit the Iceberg—Now What? -------------105

Summary -- 106

References --107

Chapter 6: Weathering the Storm---------------------- 109

Impact Bias -- 110

Implicit Bias -- 112

Hedonic Adaptation and Negativity Bias ------------114

Intentional Living: Addressing the Biases -----------115

Scarcity versus Abundance ------------------------- 117

Abundance Practices--------------------------------- 118

Importance of Gratitude: Appreciating What You Have
--120

Supporting Research for Significance of Gratitude --122

Forgiveness --124

Law of Attraction ------------------------------------125

References --128

PART III: OUTER EXCELLENCE --------------------133

Chapter 7: What is Authentic Success?--------------------135

Juxtaposing Success ----------------------------------135

Perception and Reality-------------------------------137

False Comparison ------------------------------------ 139

Aligning with Purpose ------------------------------ 141

Success in Awareness ------------------------------ 143

A Comprehensive Framework for Success ----------- 145

Recognizing the Reverse Gap and Where you Came From --- 147

Overwork or Workover! ----------------------------- 149

Summary --- 154

Further Work and Reading --------------------------- 156

References --- 156

Chapter 8: Leadership Myths Busted -------------------- 159

Spectrum of Leadership ------------------------------ 161

Emotional Awareness ------------------------------- 162

Active Listening ------------------------------------ 164

Leading Yourself ----------------------------------- 165

Historical Examples --------------------------------- 166

Summary --- 170

Further Work and Reading --------------------------- 170

References --- 171

Chapter 9: Mastering Money -------------------------- 173

Means to an End ----------------------------------- 173

Money-Time Equation ------------------------------ 175

The Right Attitude ---------------------------------- 176

The Psychology of Money ---------------------------------177

Healing Yourself --178

Money, Freedom, and Myths ----------------------------180

Visualization Techniques---------------------------------182

The Napoleon Hill Money Blueprint-------------------183

Money and Spirituality ------------------------------------185

Mending your Mindset ----------------------------- 186

Further Work and Reading--------------------------------188

References -------------------------------------- 189

PUTTING IT ALL TOGETHER: BEING THE CEO OF YOUR LIFE & HAPPINESS HYPOTHESIS--------191

Chapter 10: The CEO of Your Life ----------------------- 193

The Happiness Model -------------------------------- 194

Externalizing versus Internalizing -------------------- 195

Mastering Awareness: A Philosophical Journey----- 196

Experimenting and Developing---------------------- 197

Traditional Philosophy ------------------------------- 199

Modern Philosophy------------------------------------- 200

The CEO of Your Life ---------------------------------201

References ------------------------------------ 202

Epilogue--- 205

Acknowledgments ------------------------------------- 207

About the Authors ------------------------------------ 211

THE LEGENDARY QUEST

Preface

I AM FRANCIS YOO, a mid-career physician who, upon deep reflection, realized that becoming a doctor was never my childhood dream!

I was always interested in video games and the journeys of the main characters, which made me curious about my own journey and what it means to be truly fulfilled. Consistently, since before I entered medical school and residency, I have been pursuing and exploring philosophy, psychology, and modern and ancient Eastern and Western wisdom, along with more well-known and esoteric resources, and I have continued to do so ever since. I wanted to find a perspective that made sense to me and then use it to find authentic healing, wholeness, and fulfillment for myself and for others.

I, Ketan Kulkarni, am a mid-career physician who realized, on deep reflection, I wanted to explore beyond the traditional parameters of the practice of medicine and rekindle my passions, particularly after experiencing burnout in 2017-2018. Also, throughout my career, I have regularly encountered professionals who are unfulfilled and disgruntled, despite the fact that they always appear, superficially, to be "successful."

In my pursuit of creativity, excellence, and meaning, I have always studied and explored art, mathematics, sciences (especially theoretical physics), astrophysics, ancient and modern Eastern and Western wisdom and philosophy, psychology, mysticism, and medicine, in a comprehensive attempt to understand what living a truly successful and fulfilling life really means. I wanted to conceive a philosophy of life that makes sense to an inquisitive mind, that can be applied to life, and that can catapult anyone toward their dream life and journey. I wanted to find my own best vision and version and then help everyone else to do the same.

We two students of life met in 2019 and soon realized we were both on a quest for excellence! During our conversations, we discussed and deliberated on an array of topics. In particular, we considered the following enduring questions.

How is it that some people achieve phenomenal success? They are incredibly happy, deeply satisfied, experience the very best of human existence, live long, rich lives, enjoy a range of positive emotions, cultivate deep and gratifying relationships, embody physical vigor and vitality, undergo amazing spiritual journeys, and contribute to this world in meaningful ways, leaving a lasting and positive impact. This is observable, yet also so rare. *Why?*

Why is it that only some people seem to have it all? Is it luck? Is it simply hard work? Or does something else underpin this apparent success?

Conversely, why is it that the majority of people experience a perpetual, underlying state of discontent, distress, anxiety, worry, and stress? For most people, happiness seems to be fleeting and is often limited to vacations, weekends, gifts, and a few limited life events; for some, it is even postponed to retirement! Why do most people experience the feeling that their lives are almost constantly spiraling out of control?

Even though human beings are thinkers, and cogitation is part of our natural state, how is it that so many of us are in a constant state of hyper-analysis? Why are we overwhelmed by our own thoughts so often, as though our minds seem to have taken us over? Why do many others work themselves to death for a better future that always seems to be over the horizon?

Why do only some understand the meaning of life? Why do only some live to their full potential? Why does luck favor only some? Why do only some experience wealth? Why do only some succeed, despite so many others doing hard and smart work? What is it that determines what happens to us, our lived experience, our internal and external outcomes?

We have written this book to answer these questions, and also because we could not find a comprehensive resource that addressed these concerns in a simple, digestible format. This book is our sincere attempt to present our investigations into a variety of these fields and to describe them in a comprehensive and unified manner.

We have attempted to present a step-by-step approach that will help you, the reader, gain self-awareness, which will catapult you toward self-mastery, as you act as a catalyst in your own hero's journey, your very own Legendary Quest of life.

How to Use This Book

YOU CAN LEARN from this book by:

- Starting with introduction and then reading each chapter in sequence. You may choose not to move on to the next chapter until you have fully reflected and pondered upon the contents of each chapter.

- Reading it cover to cover first and then going back to Chapter One and taking a week or more per chapter. We suggest you intentionally apply the concepts presented in each chapter. You may choose to make your own notes for every chapter; we left space for that here or use your own journal. Many chapters contain several exercises and activities that may assist you to awaken your full potential. We suggest you fully immerse yourself and complete those exercises then store the information/notes in a safe place and refer to them in future.

- Glancing through the book, selecting a part or chapter that interests you, and then actively applying it to your life.

- Glancing through the book and reading bits and pieces that resonate with you and then actively applying those.

There is no right amount of time you need to spend reading this book. You may choose to read the book over a weekend, for instance, or take a long time mulling it over. You will know what is right for you.

You may want to periodically reread the entire book or parts of it, as you see fit and as required for you to keep applying the concepts.

You can use this book to make a small, medium, or massive difference to your life: we truly respect whatever is right for you. We are grateful for the opportunity to make a positive impact on you and your life. This book may assist in awakening you and encourage you to take massive action to realize your vision and dreams. We truly hope that book serves as a catalyst in your life's journey.

Dr. Ketan Kulkarni
Dr. Francis Yoo

Introduction

WHEN ASKED, MOST people would conclude that they are free and make autonomous decisions based on their own objective preferences. We all like to believe this assertion is true, and our experience of the world solidifies this impression. Our biological and mental systems combine to give us the experience that all of our choices are rational.

To give an example, a heroin addict often believes that his or her choices are perfectly natural. Perhaps there are moments of self-awareness interspersed with the suffering and delusion, but when the profound biological need for heroin arises, then many addicts will experience the sensation that taking heroin will solve all of their problems. They will absolutely prioritize this, at the expense of anything and everything else, no matter how bad their life gets. An outsider will immediately recognize the obvious sadness inherent in this, but sometimes the addict can never break out of this compulsive behavior and simply does not survive.

This is an unusually extreme example, but, in principle it's not too different from the reality of many people's lives. The addict has created a mental model based on false priorities, which leads to errant behavior. Most of our behavior never becomes that errant. But many of us do, indeed, spend our lives within a model that dictates our behavior to a great extent. If we are able to take a step back and view the situation dispassionately, as with the heroin addict, then we can recognize this and take action. But too many of us plow on regardless, following the same reductive patterns from cradle to grave, and consequently, we never experience true fulfillment.

In the course of our practice, professional lives, and investigation, we authors have developed a mental model that outlines how most humans spend most of their time. This model is based on a vast amount of evidence from diverse sources, including (but not limited to) study of ancient wisdom, contemporary evidence, psychoanalysis, scientific research, and quantum physics. We recognize that we, ourselves, have spent countless hours in this model over the course of our personal and professional lives. In retrospect, this model has been the singular driving force, even during major crises and life events in our own life journeys.

There are a multitude of factors that feed into this mental model, but the outcome is largely uniform for most people: we ultimately find ourselves pursuing patterns of behavior that are limiting and even self-destructive. Not, perhaps, as self-destructive as living on the streets, shooting up heroin. But debilitating enough in their own way. We believe this is a grotesque waste of human potential. We also believe that addressing this undesirable situation will not only be beneficial for people as individuals, but will also result in a vastly improved society.

But in order to achieve this, we first need to understand the model itself:

The Limited-Self Model

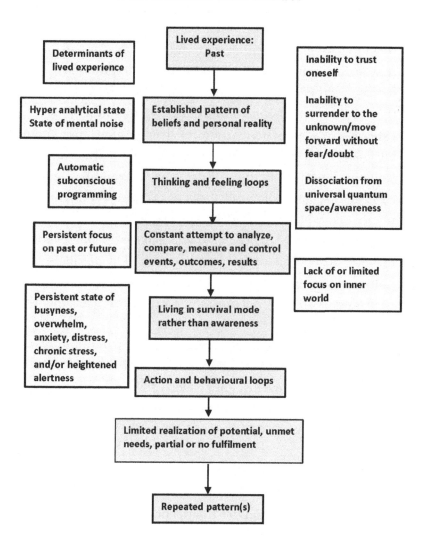

Why are Most People Unfulfilled?

This model is a manifestation of a limited self. Most people reside within this construct in all aspects of their lives.

Most people are stuck in a state of hyper-analysis; they are drowning in their own thoughts and emotions. They cannot seem to dissociate themselves from this state of mental noise that seems to drive them all the time. In addition, most of us focus on either our past or our future and rarely, if ever, on the present moment. The majority of human beings experience a persistent state of background discontent, busyness, anxiety, overwhelm, stress, heightened alertness, or some form of distress most of the time. They do not seem to be able to separate themselves from this visceral discontent, no matter what happens. Happiness and joy seem to be fleeting and limited to brief moments such as holidays, certain life events, and sporadic circumstances. The result is that individuals believe these states are normal and expected! That they must exist! And that life is but a struggle, not a wonderful journey.

Many things, including our childhood, parenting, peers, media, Internet, culture, geography, society, politics, major and minor life events, our successes and failures and emotional experiences combine to craft our lived experience. Even if we have long forgotten about these determinants, they shape us.

Most people allow the lived experience from their pasts to establish a pattern of beliefs and personal reality in the present, which then dictates their behavior in the future. This creates thinking and feeling loops (repetitive and often redundant patterns), which results in continual attempts to (i) analyze, compare, measure and (ii) control events, outcomes, and results in life. Most people do not even realize that these patterns have become compulsive! The resultant programming of their subconscious mind further feeds into this and strengthens these patterns.

At this point, people are living in survival mode (as if just trying to catch a breath), rather than in a state of awareness. And it's at this point in the model that this state of mind feeds into reductive behavioral loops, actions, and decisions. Ultimately, this results in the limited realization of potential, in unmet needs, and in severely limited fulfillment. This pattern then repeats, forming a highly undesirable and self-destructive circle. Remember the heroin addict example?

The sensory reality of this pattern results in an inability to trust one's self. Once this inability becomes cemented, there is then also an inability to move forward in life without feeling fear and doubt, underpinned by an inability to surrender to the unknown. This then creates a dissociation from universal and quantum awareness, meaning people become dissociated from their inner worlds. So many people feel disconnected, both form themselves and from other human beings!

Ultimately, the consequence of this is that people are unable to connect with their authentic selves, with their true desires and motivations in life, and this can result in them pursuing paths that are unedifying, paths that do not fulfill them. The outcome of this is that people feel dissatisfied no matter how much they achieve and accrue; and yet, due to the model outlined above, they cannot recognize this aberrant thinking and behavior.

Rather than break free from these unhealthy patterns of behavior, people, instead, tend to believe, if they work harder at chasing some illusory goals, they will somehow fill the hole inside of themselves. However, this hole never seems to be satiated. It merely persists and expands as they keep ploughing forward.

But this is all a total delusion. The situation will never change, any more than the situation of a heroin addict will change by acquiring more heroin. Only by connecting with the authentic self, developing a healthy and productive mental model, and making progress toward achieving fulfilling and genuine personal goals will the situation improve.

It is thus essential to get on the right path as soon as possible. We cannot emphasize this enough. As long as you're operating within the reductive mental model described above, you are critically limiting yourself as a human being. You are hamstringing yourself, condemning your life to being one of gnawing dissatisfaction and unfulfilled potential. You will indeed never fulfill your true potential until you connect with your authentic self. Essentially, you're going to be unhappy unless you address this. Or, in a best-case scenario, you will be less happy than is actually possible.

This is why we have written this book. To try to help people understand where they are going wrong in life, and to help them connect with their authentic selves, so they can unleash their true potential. It is never too late or too early to achieve this. But it is important to get yourself on the road to success and happiness as soon as possible.

In this book, we're going to discuss the factors that tend to separate each of us from our authentic selves. We will explain how to become more self-aware and connect with this authentic aspect of ourselves. And we will outline a blueprint for how to achieve success on your terms, so you're the CEO of your own life. We will subsequently share a happiness model, which is the polar opposite of the self-limiting variant included in this introduction.

Above all else, we want people to come away from this book feeling and understanding that anything is possible. But it's only possible if we master our true selves first. And the first step in this process is for us to understand why so many of us are separated from our authentic selves and focused on pursuing inauthentic goals.

NOTES

_____

_____

_____

_____

_____

_____

_____

_____

_____

_____

_____

_____

_____

_____

PART I

RECOGNIZING THE PROBLEM

Chapter 1

Are You Pursuing Authentic Goals?

The Irony

ONE OF THE IRONIC things about our social systems and wider society is that modern education can be one of the most reductive experiences in our lives. This certainly isn't something we tend to hear discussed in the media or promoted generally. And thus, consequently, it's not a perspective most of the population is familiar with or that they particularly embrace.

But what often happens during education, especially in the lower grades, is the potential of young people is essentially limited. Young people's possibilities are throttled from an early age. Indeed, how many young people ultimately end up pursuing their real dreams? The answer is it's only a small percentage, as students are effectively told during their schooling what they can reasonably aspire to do and become.

Albert Einstein was told often during his school years that he would not amount to much of anything in his life! The rest is history...

But that's just the start of the process. Everything children become familiar with at school—the structure, the hierarchy, the authority, the system of rules—is then mirrored by employment and the labor market. More and more restrictions are layered on top of them, until most people effectively lose the will to chase what they really want. They end up trying to squeeze themselves into a narrow mold of possibility. The parameters of their existence are effectively narrowed, until they can't even see the potential of their own existence.

What happens to most people in this oppressive system is that they literally lose their own self-identity, or, in many cases, it never even develops in the first place. A fundamental aspect of this is that many people never develop a clear picture of what they want, because they allow external projections to control the way they think. They are told what is possible for them. This is driven home to them every day, in institutionalized settings, and, consequently, they come to believe this is reality.

This is such a tragedy, as no one is born with such limitations. This outcome is simply a product of (social) conditioning. Modern education is a compelling example of this, but there are many other factors at play, as well, including the influence of media, culture, peer pressure and wider social examples. To a very great extent, most people ultimately live a proscribed existence whose parameters are defined by a combination of some, and usually all, of these influences.

The natural consequence of this is that people never explore their potential. But there are other, less obvious negative consequences, as well.

Success that Becomes No Success

One of the most compelling consequences is that successes don't turn out to be successes! This sounds like a nonsensical statement, but, in reality, it is surprisingly common.

Many people grow up with a constrained concept of what represents success. This is understandable, as the society, peer, culture, and media pump out a distinct image of success almost relentlessly. Thus, it's only natural that people are drawn to this image and begin to pursue it, believing that happiness will result when they achieve it.

Unfortunately, this doesn't happen, as success is a personal journey. There are as many versions of success as there are people. So, when you follow someone else's version of success, you don't ultimately feel successful when you have achieved it, because you are pursuing a dream that isn't yours in the first place. This is why self-knowledge is so important in the process of becoming successful; it's only then that you can confidently pursue an authentic path through life.

One of the intriguing aspects of our measurements of success is that they are almost always quantitative and external. Furthermore, it's important to note how modern society generally places little or no emphasis on internal feelings, particularly in the Western world. We still acquiesce with this state of being, and we absolutely submit to the prevailing culture, but there is nonetheless a strong force of coercion exhibited by the powerful forces mentioned previously—education, media, social example.

Our Measures of Success are Flawed

On one level, focusing on the external, the quantitative, makes perfect sense. It is simply easier to measure how much of something exists. But the reality is that success is both quantitative and qualitative. You cannot simply say, "This person has x amount of money and y amount of status; therefore, they are more successful and more fulfilled than this other person who has less!"

A classic example of this would be the person who chooses to buy a plot of land, grows their own food, subsists, and is completely self-reliant, while being in touch with nature every day. People are living this way all over the world. They may have no particular wealth, no particular net worth, yet they may feel happier and more fulfilled than many people who are billionaires. That's because they chose their own specific and authentic path through life and so are now experiencing success on their own terms, not on someone else's terms.

There is another interesting aspect of this that is particularly important. Often, the process of achieving success and fulfillment is not a linear journey. There are problems along the way; there are obstacles along the way. It can take quite some time before you veer, seemingly accidentally, onto the right path. You might have to fail several times in order to become successful, although these experiences should always be viewed as life lessons rather than failures.

And the people who really succeed from this process are those who retain what could be described as an inner child. They are driven by enthusiasm, by very pure motives. A good example here would be Thomas Edison, who strived endlessly in order to become the revolutionary inventor he undoubtedly was. What sustained Edison was the unadulterated enthusiasm for what he was doing, the honest human desire that overrode societal programming.

Interestingly, Edison didn't receive a huge amount of training. He was very much an autodidact.[1] In short, he didn't go through all of the systems described previously. While formal education can undoubtedly be valuable and can set you on the correct path for your life, it can also be just another stepping stone on a preordained life path. It can narrow both your view of possibility and the potential for your existence.

What Do You Really Want?

And the key takeaway here isn't to focus on what you're doing wrong. The important thing is to focus on what you really want. Your heart's desire could indeed be a fairly stereotypical version of success. But it has to be an authentic version of this, one that suits your particular values.

This can only be achieved through self-knowledge; only when you truly know and understand yourself can you pursue your own authentic life journey. Many people believe they are doing this already but are, in fact, pursuing goals defined by external forces.

A valuable way to begin to understand this is via the Enneagram of Personality.[2] This is a model of the human psyche that is principally understood and taught as a typology of nine interconnected personality types. The Enneagram defines nine personality types (sometimes referred to as "enneatypes"), which are represented by the points on a geometric figure, known as an enneagram, that indicate connections between the types. Thus, there can be overlap between personality types, with each individual manifesting different aspects of various personality types.

One interesting aspect of the Enneagram model is that different personality types can arrive at similar behaviors via different fundamental motivations and quirks, which may not be immediately obvious. For example, a Type Three personality, the achiever, is driven to accumulate a list of accomplishments. A healthy Type Three will understand that they have inherent value, whereas an unhealthy Type Three will feel they have limited value. So, the former can add value to their lives as a human being, while the latter will feel compelled to pursue a list of accomplishments in order to fill this perceived chasm of worth.

The key here is that you can still be very productive, hugely driven, and get a lot of things done. But if you're not well-adjusted and grounded in healthy values, you will find yourself ultimately doing things for the wrong reasons, and you won't attain the authentic fulfillment we've already spoken about. Whereas a healthy Type Three will know that they have this inherent value, so their focus is never on increasing this; instead, their inner fire will drive them to do things to increase their happiness and sense of fulfillment. That will then make them feel better about themselves and help to create a virtuous circle of positive behavior.

Thus, two people can follow similar paths and have a lot of overlap in personality types, but their behavior can emanate from completely different aspects of motivation. So, everyone needs to understand when they are pursuing a certain path through life, and indeed, when they have so much energy and drive in a certain direction, whether they truly desire the outcomes and will feel fulfillment from them. Or, instead, whether they're seeking some form of external gratification, or the achievements associated with this task will merely serve the superficial purpose of buttressing their lack of self-esteem.

We are Submerged in a Matrix

It's also important to know that it's difficult to understand one's self. There are so many external influences on our lives, and we now live in a 24/7 media and technology matrix.

With the advent of smartphones, a lot of people are constantly absorbing media. We live in a figurative media bubble. This can make it extremely difficult to drill down to the authentic self, as we are so influenced by the external messaging we receive from our constant attachment to media.

Also, psychology isn't in stasis. Our personal psychology can even fluctuate from one moment to another, so understanding what motivates us and discovering the appropriate authentic journey for our own lives do not necessarily make for a straightforward process. This is where awareness, emotional intelligence, and self-knowledge come in. We will be discussing these critical concepts later in the book.

But this concept of the authentic journey governs so much of our existence. All of our life decisions are effectively governed by this, and it's only through developing self-knowledge that you'll be able to recognise this. For example, someone could desire a particular car, as they've always been passionate about motor vehicles or require a certain form of transportation for their family. This would be an example of an authentic reason to purchase something. Conversely, another person could want the same car, but it is because they were triggered by a neighbor owning a certain vehicle or someone at work, or because they see a particular commercial and are convinced it would be a good idea and make them somehow a better person. (Indeed, car ads usually focus on precisely this!) Needless to say, the latter example would be an inauthentic reason to purchase a motor vehicle.

The Dichotomy of Choices

This dichotomy feeds into so many of our life choices. And it is probably no more specifically manifested than in our work and life ambitions.

That drive is a good thing in the workplace and our working lives is almost perpetually communicated to us. And that's not necessarily untrue. It's just ultimately inadequate.

What is really important is *directed* drive. While someone completely lacking in motivation and drive can certainly lead to a lack of happiness and fulfillment, drive without direction can equally lead people down an unending cul-de-sac of misery.

Thus, we have all witnessed people in life who seem to be hugely motivated. They seem to work extremely hard and are ostensibly successful. They have the material trappings of success, and on the surface of it, they have achieved what is often described as the American Dream. They may genuinely believe they are taking the right path through life. But their focus may be so squarely set on achievement, they can be completely lacking in self-awareness of their actual authentic desires.

Yet such people often ultimately crash. They reach a point where they can't push themselves any longer, and then they wonder what the point of all that effort has been. Has what they have achieved and accumulated resulted in happiness and fulfillment? In many cases, the answer is negative, because they were never pursuing their authentic goals in the first place. They have instead been exhibiting behaviors that are completely driven by external factors. They have never followed their own hearts or pursued their own dreams, and consequently, they ultimately end up with an empty feeling, even after having achieved what appears to be tangible success. This is the textbook basis for a midlife crisis, which then sends a person's life careening off in another unwanted and unhealthy direction.

Look Within Not Without

It's important in this process that people indeed identify this within themselves. People can be guided onto the right path, but they must choose to take that journey themselves. It is not something someone else can choose for you, no matter how qualified they may be. If you don't have this quality of self-knowledge, you won't acquire the end goal you ultimately desire.

And that goal can differ hugely for different people. We shouldn't place one ideal on a pedestal and assert that everyone should aim for this particular outcome. Not everyone wants to add meaningful value to the entire world; that is not the goal of their distinct life journey. Maybe they want to add value to their family or their local community or some other aspect of their lives. Or maybe they wish to produce art or some manifestation of things they need to express or want to participate in a nonprofit organization or help people less fortunate than themselves.

The core desires can vary widely, both in quality and quantity. The important thing is that no one should be diminished for this. We should instead recognise that everyone needs to pursue their own authentic goals.

There are countless examples of this that could be cited. But one that comes to mind in particular is that of Jill. She was a highly successful businesswoman who was making $400,000 a year at age forty. Materially and in terms of success, she seemed to have it all. But you shouldn't judge a book by its cover!

Jill was working eighty hours every week, in an attempt to climb the corporate ladder. Yet she had failed to address some of her critical needs. She longed for a loving relationship but never had the time to actually seek one. She ignored many advances from friends and colleagues, because her inclination was always to "get through" this promotion or this job, and then she would think about it. But the treadmill never stops. Now, she feels she has enough money, but her previous friends have moved on and settled with their families. She finds herself feeling quite lonely and has taken up drinking in an attempt to numb this feeling. She wonders whether all of this endeavor was worth it, in the end.

There are many lessons we can take from this example and information, but one of the most important is to never delay our happiness. Pursuing our most important and authentic goals should always be our life priority. This is not something to set aside until retirement. It's not something to even set aside until tomorrow. We never know what tomorrow will bring, so there is no better time than the present to begin the process of following our hearts.

Many people learn this lesson the hard way. For example, one of our acquaintance's wives, the most senior business woman in the community, was planning to retire in two years and travel all over the world. A very common life goal, of course. This woman had worked extremely hard all of her life to build up a nest egg, so she could enjoy her golden years. Another extremely common life plan. But there was a problem. She contracted metastatic pancreatic cancer and likely will not live even until next year.

This could happen to any one of us. We think we will definitely get eighty to ninety years to cram in everything we want to do. But it doesn't necessarily work that way. A friend of ours was dating a younger woman. During the relationship, she became ill with cancer. She battled against the condition for six months, and it looked for a while as if she had a promising prognosis. But unfortunately, she took a turn for the worse and ultimately passed away. This was a healthy and relatively young woman; indeed, she was only thirty-four!

Universal Myth: I'll be Happy When...

The common cultural trope is that you work your entire life with this exalted goal of retirement always on the horizon.

But this is one of the greatest myths and mistakes anyone could ever make. Postponing your happiness, postponing your success, postponing the pursuit of your dreams is always a massive error. This shouldn't be something you view on the distant horizon. It should be every day of your life. It should be the fundamental focus of your existence. You could describe this process as "working retirement." You should be constantly retired and also constantly pursuing your goals!

Thus, retirement isn't a carrot that continually dangles tantalizingly out of your reach. It should be a priority, a state of mind, life, and being, that you seek to achieve as quickly as possible. You have to live with contentment all of the time, as you could lose your life at any moment. And even if you do live to a ripe old age, you will encounter life challenges along the way. So, make sure you're doing what your heart desires today!

It is important to note here that we are not referring to *instant gratification*. Instant gratification refers to a temptation, an urge to need or want something and then a tendency to forego larger future benefits in order to obtain an immediate, albeit smaller, benefit. While we all have needs, desires, or experiences that we want to satisfy in a timely manner, surrendering fully to a hedonistic, instant-gratification lifestyle does not lead to lasting happiness and satisfaction. We will address this fully in future chapters.

Another physician colleague of ours has enjoyed an extremely successful clinical career. He has worked phenomenally hard and now has a net worth of approximately $5o million, a financial position of which most people would be envious. But there's a catch. He has worked in practice for forty-three years, from dawn to dusk most of this period. He's an intelligent person, and he's invested well. But you could argue he has absolutely no wisdom!

Because now, when he was seventy-nine years old, Covid hit. Suddenly, what is the point of having $5o million? You can't go anywhere or do anything! He possibly doesn't have long left; he is not as strong, fit, or energetic as in his youth. So, all he is going to do is pass this money down to the children. His kids, not surprisingly, have had outstanding educations, are all doctors, and don't need the money! He wonders what to do next. He wonders how he can find a larger purpose and make meaningful contributions to society at large.

This is a person whom we can hugely admire in many ways. Undoubtedly, someone who has a work ethic and drive to be envied. An intelligent, credentialed, qualified, and successful person. Yet, if we were to assess him harshly, he has effectively wasted his life. He has never pursued his own authentic goals. He has profoundly postponed his own happiness for some future that never arrived. This is a cast-iron example of precisely what you shouldn't do!

This mentality of postponing our happiness pervades our entire culture, particularly financially. We're always saving up for a rainy day that never comes. People are taught to max out their 401K policies and make sure that they save up diligently for this retirement, which is always looming enticingly on the horizon. It is almost heretical to go against this mentality, it is so ingrained. People are never taught in terms of pursuing their authenticity. They are instead taught in terms of what works, societally.

But this is a completely false form of prudence. It's instead much more prudent to enjoy what you have today and to reap what you sow while you're still in a position to benefit from it. In short, your golden years should be right now!

References

1. National Park Service. (2015). *Edison Biography.*
2. Owens, M. (2021). *What is the Enneagram of Personality?*

NOTES

_____

_____

_____

_____

_____

_____

_____

_____

_____

_____

_____

_____

_____

_____

_____

_____

Chapter 2

Too Entitled for Your Title

What Determines Well-being?

IN 1938, A GROUP of scientists began tracking the health of Harvard sophomores. The Great Depression had been a trying time for the United States, and it was hoped that this longitudinal study would reveal critical information on how to lead healthy and happy lives.

Eighty years on, the Harvard Study of Adult Development has proved to be instrumental in our understanding of human well-being.[1] And perhaps the biggest, and most distinct, takeaway from the research is that the quality of relationships we experience has a powerful influence on our general state of health. It is commonly known that taking care of our bodies is important, but data from the Harvard research suggests that tending to our relationships is perhaps equally critical.

In fact, close relationships not only help to delay mental and physical decline, but they are also better predictors of longevity than social class, IQ, or even genetics. As the study was expanded, it was found that this proved true across both Harvard graduates and inter-city participants. Several studies have since identified that feeling a sense of satisfaction with relationships at age fifty has been a better predictor of physical health than physical factors such as cholesterol levels.[2]

This is a critical pillar of understanding when we begin to craft what our definition of success will look like. As we've discussed previously, everyone has their own version of success, and there definitely isn't a one-size-fits-all definition of this concept. But good health and physical outcomes are surely fundamental to this definition. This cannot be achieved without these two key factors: strong relationships and a distinctive and self-aware direction in life.

It's Not About the Labels

In order to achieve this, we really need to drill down efficiently into the core of what motivates us. This is tremendously difficult to do, as there are so many external influences on our psyche, which is why self-awareness is so important. But one of the keys is not to pursue goals because they project a certain image of what is deemed to be success, and instead to pursue them because they instead will authentically improve our lives.

Labels play a vital role in this process. As we both work in the medical field, we frequently encounter doctors who are somewhat fixated with their titles, i.e., with being Dr. Johnson and the kudos that redound from that. In fact, this is quite normal within the medical profession. But does this really lead to happiness? Does being so attached to a title actually lead to fulfillment?

Effectively, being able to be called a doctor, and being able to use that as part of your name, is seen as a manifestation or measurement of what society deems to be "success." It is recognized as an achievement or accomplishment. But, in and of itself, it is completely meaningless! Authentic happiness and success aren't associated with these titles, as the Harvard study demonstrates. Ultimately, attaining respect from people you may not know or who don't matter to you will have almost no impact on your happiness, fulfillment, health, or sense of well-being. So, prioritizing that over authentic goals that will positively influence these critical aspects of your life makes absolutely no sense whatsoever!

Thus, it's important to understand that your title is ultimately a particularly poor way to measure your success. This is deeply ironic, as we inherently associate success with certain recognizable titles. It is almost automatically assumed that someone working as a doctor, lawyer, scientist, or one of the many other traditionally middle-class professions, is successful. Indeed, it is often automatically assumed that they are happy and fulfilled, as well, although perhaps at least our assessment of this aspect of life has become slightly more sophisticated and nuanced.

We Have Got It Wrong and Continue to Do So

But even though we have established that there is more to human fulfillment than simply occupying a certain station in life, it remains something society pushes us into from a very early age. Even the people who care most about us will tend to promote this.

How many people became physicians, barristers, accountants, politicians, and indeed pursued many other bourgeois life goals, simply because their parents advocated it, almost from the moment they first tasted their mother's milk? And how many of these people ended up deeply unsatisfied yet still pursued that path, because they thought it was what they were supposed to do?

The answer is that it's all too many. It's millions and millions of people. And if there is one thing that has become abundantly clear in our investigation of the human psyche and well-being, it is that failing to pursue your own authentic goals based on your true self will never result in fulfillment. You may have a bearable existence, you may experience fleeting moments of happiness, you may create memories that you genuinely treasure. But there will still be a fundamental emptiness at the core of your being, as you never satisfied your desires, your dreams, and your purpose for being on this planet in the first place.

What will typically happen in this scenario is the unfulfilled person will seek more success as a substitute for the pursuit of their real goals. In short, as we've discussed previously, they will seek a quantitative solution to the problem, rather than a qualitative solution. But this is more likely to exacerbate the issue, as opposed to addressing it.

Need of a Comprehensive Framework for Success: Don't Miss the Forest for the Trees

So, if we are to achieve our own personal version of success, we have to recognize not only what success is, but also what it definitely is not! This is where self-awareness needs to be factored into the equation. But we also need to fundamentally understand that we should never be living another person's version of success, in order to satisfy or impress others. There is another fundamental dichotomy here between internalizing and externalizing. We have to learn to listen to the internal mechanisms that guide us on whether or not we're successful, rather than focus just on external manifestations of success.

In the medical field, we encounter many examples of this precise phenomenon. You could argue that the title, *Doctor*, is the most sought-after of all. It is certainly something that can generate pride in households all over the world and is almost by definition seen as being a symbol of success. Consequently, many people working in the medical field have ultimately followed this life goal due to external pressures; they essentially sleepwalk through their lives, complying with someone else's impression of how they should exist.

It's quite common to encounter doctors who have effectively spent more than thirty years in the same room! What could possibly be more limiting than this existence? Naturally, they have accrued a creditable level of proficiency in that particular field, and they have achieved something rather rare in proportional terms across the population as a whole. Furthermore, most doctors have also experienced a decent level of financial success. These are all nice things to have, but even collectively, they do not necessarily add up to an authentic or fulfilling existence.

We have had the opportunity to meet with many medical professionals at conferences and other social events across the globe. It is extremely common to encounter people within our profession who have allowed their own lives to spiral out of control. That might sound like an exaggeration, but it certainly is not! All too common are the tales of the doctor who has allowed himself or herself to be shoehorned into a particular position, possibly a division or department head, and now they're sequestered in endless meetings. There is a bigger workload, their hours seem to have multiplied, and they often end up in these positions because no one else will do it! They are frequently displeased, don't feel in control, and are cynical. Meanwhile, real life is passing them by outside, with their own lives irrevocably severed from all that is organic and real.

So, when you find yourself in that situation, when you begin to have the gnawing sensation that life is passing you by and you're missing out on enriching life experiences…, do you really think that being able to call yourself a doctor properly compensates for this? I completely missed out on life, but occasionally I get to tell people that I'm a doctor, and they're moderately impressed for a few seconds… *Hmm…* Not really a massive form of compensation, is it?

Burn-in Not Burn-out

The key to life is finding a healthy balance between authenticity and the pursuit of external goals. If you tilt the seesaw too decisively in one direction, your life will teeter precariously.

One interesting example here is the science-fiction writer Philip K Dick, unquestionably one of the greatest narrative writers in his genre and arguably one of the most insightful pure-prose writers ever. In terms of authenticity, Dick lived the ideal existence. He absolutely believed in what he was doing from a creative perspective, and he committed himself to his calling with absolute abandon. On the flip side, he lived in total destitution for most of his existence, had a particularly chaotic personal life, often experienced poor health, and then died just as he was getting successful, having been penniless for most of his life. This feeds into the Japanese concept of *Ikigai*, having a direction or purpose in life that provides fulfillment and meaning.

When we look back at the life of Dick today, we can judge it to have been a massive success. Several of his books have been made into films, and the influence of his thematic preoccupations has been truly profound. Dick was a true auteur, light years ahead of his time, who left a literary legacy that few people will ever match. Equally, the actual living of Dick's life was probably not particularly enjoyable! His writing was obviously an escape from his living circumstances, which were often impoverished. This is a highly extreme payoff between authenticity and achievement.

Certainly, the vast majority of people will want to strike a more palatable balance between the two.

Nonetheless, if anyone creates a list of successful people, it will be tangibly tailored toward the qualities that have influenced them in life. Almost inevitably, you will see figures such as writers, artists, musicians, psychologists, philosophers, inventors, sportspeople, and other inspirational figures who have achieved something of particular note and effectively changed the direction of human life or thought. It will be very rare to see someone on the list primarily due to their net worth.

So, that's a very important life lesson in itself. But this exercise to identify who you think are successful people enables you to determine who is fundamentally successful from your personal perspective. This can be very informative and can provide a real insight into a suitable life direction based on your priorities.

Bring in the Dollars!

Interestingly, if you encounter people who place their sole life focus on their financial worth, they are almost without exception unhappy! And this is completely regardless of the level of "success" they attain. In our lives, we have encountered several prolific real estate developers, probably worth more than $100 million, and yet most of them are noticeably unhappy. They don't talk to anybody, they don't experience connection with other people, and they don't radiate any form of joy about life. Isn't this a terrible waste?

You will also find that people in the entrepreneurial fields will never just focus on their specific area of work. For example, doctors tend to define themselves as being doctors, or they might specifically indicate they're gastroenterologists or plastic surgeons, or that they work in some other specific discipline. Same with people in finance, the legal profession, and other areas we typically consider to be high-ranking, serious, and credible.

That doesn't apply to entrepreneurs. They will provide a much more open-ended assessment of what they do in life. This then tends to translate into a more organic and open-minded lifestyle in terms of what is possible. They are focusing on adding value and making a meaningful contribution rather than solely pursuing monetary benefits or a particular title.

What About the Workaholic?

Ultimately, from our experience, we would argue that most people who are actually authentically successful and happy, at least as we would define it, are not particularly tied to their professional title or any of the trappings associated with their profession. Their professional work, in fact, is a relatively small part of their lives, and it facilitates their overall existence rather than be their sole focus. Again, it comes back to that concept of balance, and creating the ideal balance between authenticity and achievement is critical for virtually every person.

It can be argued that some people are so driven, they simply must work ninety hours every week and constantly chase achievements and success. But are they really expressing their authentic selves? Are they chasing those achievements and successes for the right reasons? And will they ultimately end up being fulfilled? We would suggest the answers to those questions are *no, no,* and *no*!

The Double-edged Digital World

It's also important to emphasize that this mentality of being attached to a title may have made some sense in the past due to inflexible hierarchical systems. We would still argue that it wasn't entirely ideal, but it at least correlated with the economic reality of life in the pre-Internet age. Today, it is a relic, a dinosaur, an irrelevance!

You don't have to live such a prescribed existence nowadays. The Web has opened up a planet of possibility to anyone with an open mind. This makes the preoccupation with titles completely meaningless, along with the supposed esteem in the eyes of others. The world of information and technology has already proven to be far more versatile than rigid traditional structures, while also offering people a degree of flexibility that enables them to pursue their true authenticity.

Ironically, the Internet is a double-edged sword. The nature of its now hugely social media-driven culture is that people do, indeed, end up seeking external validation from others. Too many people are chasing clicks and likes and feedback, when they should instead be pursuing more authentic goals. It may have a different flavor, but this is still the same trap as being too heavily associated with your title.

You're valuing something because of its impact on others, rather than its impact on your own life.

Social media and other platforms, which can be positive both personally and professionally, shouldn't be entirely disregarded. But when you're engaging with the sole purpose of building an image in the minds of others, so they will respond to you in a certain way, you have veered decisively away from the course of authenticity. This will only cause you problems at a later date, as you either become too addicted to attention and it comes to define you, or else you'll experience a mini-crisis when you realize you've been pursuing goals that fail to nurture your well-being. To say nothing of the negativity and abuse you're likely to encounter on social platforms, if you spend too much time engaging with them.

Old Dogs Can't Learn New Tricks... Or Can They?

This also applies to people who follow a more traditional path through life, aggressively chasing titles and conventional signifiers of "success." Typically, they will experience a midlife crisis. They will begin to sense the grave looming on the horizon, and they will realize, as we've been discussing in this chapter, that they have effectively wasted their lives! They haven't had the moral and intellectual courage required to question who they are, and, consequently, they have allowed themselves to be pigeonholed into a marketer's idea of success and fulfillment.

They then feel remorse at the time wasted and also feel trapped in terms of seeking a new direction. They're old dogs who don't know how to teach themselves new tricks. The title and position that have restricted them have also come to define them, and they don't know how to break out of these roles.

As Andy Dufresne commented in *The Shawshank Redemption*, we have a simple choice in life: get busy living, or get busy dying. People in this situation recognize they are effectively busy dying, but they do not know how to get busy living, as they've never taken the time to develop the apparatus required.

The key is to move the *Titanic* before it hits the iceberg! To identify and set out on your authentic life path in time to minimize any regret you may otherwise encounter. And to remain flexible, to guard against cognitive rigidity.

There is one final concept that most professional people will encounter at some point. Things may be progressing swimmingly in their career, they may have found a life path and goal that suits their authentic selves, and they may have accumulated enough wealth to purchase a nice house and car and to afford a relatively lavish lifestyle.

But it can then become quite easy at this point to stop challenging yourself and just to accept what you have already achieved. To begin to go through the motions. You're in a position of privilege, so you cease searching for the real goals and journey that is always burning within you. In short, you're in a comfort zone. And a comfort zone can feel comfortable for a while, but it can ultimately be quite limiting.

Thus, maintaining a growth mindset at all times during your life and career is important, as is defining this notion of growth in the right way. It's not just about growing your net worth, developing your wealth, and expanding your success in quantitative terms. It is also about growing your quality of life, nurturing your experiences, and ensuring that your outlook and behavior continue to evolve in line with your mindset.

This is far more liberating and healthier than allowing your title to define who you are.

References

1. Harvard Health Publishing. (2017). *The secret to happiness? Here's some advice from the longest-running study on happiness.*

2. The Harvard Gazette. (2017). *Good genes are nice, but joy is better.*

NOTES

_____

_____

_____

_____

_____

_____

_____

_____

_____

_____

_____

_____

_____

Chapter 3

Your Core Beliefs are Wrong

YOUR CORE BELIEFS about success, wealth, and money are wrong, at least most of the time. And it's not your fault!

This is ironic, because you probably have a very clear image in your mind of what success looks like, as well as what will be required to achieve it. When we think about success, we immediately associate a sense of struggle with the process.

How else can you achieve success, without investing endless hours of sheer effort? You have to burn the midnight oil, negotiate the obstacles, peaks, and troughs that are inevitable, and show a huge amount of fortitude.

Success is Slow and Hard... Or Is It?

That is the impression most people have of any form of success. But it's not necessarily the reality. The core belief, that you require immense will, discipline, and perseverance in order to achieve success, is not necessarily well-founded. Some people become multimillionaires almost overnight, especially in the digital world. Perhaps they launch an app or have a particular breakthrough that ultimately leads to their financial success.

In some cases, success comes quite easily, without the need for making massive sacrifices. It really depends on the situation. There are countless examples of people who achieve an inordinate degree of success virtually overnight. Some of the most successful people in business and the arts went from being completely unknown to achieving phenomenal success in an extremely short period of time.

There are so many examples of this. One that immediately comes to mind is J.K. Rowling. The author of the *Harry Potter* books is now a mega-success. But that couldn't have been more removed from her position when she began writing. Essentially, she was a penniless single mother.[1] While she certainly invested an amount of time in her work and also experienced rejection, when success came, it escalated unbelievably rapidly. Her books quickly went viral, Hollywood was soon knocking on the door, and she was absolutely made for life within a matter of months. This all came from after the short period of time, while she was in receipt of welfare, when Rowling concentrated on writing.

Similarly, there have been many overnight millionaires in the world of technology, with the likes of Mark Zuckerberg and Bill Gates experiencing massive success in a relatively short time frame. No doubt they would argue that they worked hard in order to acquire their computing skills, and there is, of course, some degree of truth in that assertion. But the actual success that led to their wealth and security didn't require a vast amount of time or plausibly excruciating effort.

Zuckerberg's Facebook project caught fire during college; he rapidly became a multimillionaire and, eventually, a billionaire. Gates was a billionaire within ten years of dropping out of Harvard and within five years of first approaching IBM regarding software. [2] That's how quickly massive success can happen. Similar examples can be found in sports, music, the movie industry, and many other fields.

This goes against the grain of our general impression of success. Most people's core belief is that you have to slog your guts out and virtually kill yourself in order to be very successful. Many other people believe that you cannot have it all, that you have to sacrifice something in order to possess something else. It's almost like a seesaw, where it is impossible for both sides to be in a lofty position simultaneously. Something has to give, right?

Long Hours Culture

But that's not true. There are numerous examples of people who do have everything they could wish for materially, but have also managed to maintain a core balance to their lives. And life is all about balance—your own version of that balance, to be precise! If you don't strike something near to an appropriate balance between work and recreation, there is no doubt you will suffer mentally, psychologically, and eventually physically. The evidence supporting that is crystal clear.

For example, a meta-analysis of scientific studies, authored by Wong, Chan, and Ngan and published in the *International Journal of Environmental Research and Public*

KETAN KULKARNI & FRANCIS YOO

Health, concluded that "employees working long hours were vulnerable to suffering from diverse types of occupational health problems," emphasizing the deleterious effects of long working hours on occupational health."[3]

Yet often we are given the opposite impression. That success is about obsession. About concentrating with almost superhuman intensity on achievement at the expense of absolutely everything else in your life. This is certainly the picture painted in much of popular and prevailing media. And, generally speaking, there is an obsession with people who are super-wealthy. But the question is never asked whether these people are, in fact, happy and functioning human beings.

In fact, precisely because of that lack of balance, often the super-rich are extremely unhappy people. They seem to have everything, but this is a seductive illusion. It's extremely easy to be rich and unhappy, rich and burned out, and even rich and lonely.

You would think, logically, that someone with a huge amount of money would experience a wealth of social opportunities, and this certainly can be the case. But many super-wealthy people simply don't place any value in nurturing personal relationships, and consequently they don't develop meaningful social connections. They become the stereotypical workaholics, forever fretting over something that will ultimately have absolutely no impact on their lives, while everything that would nurture and fulfill them is neglected and actually exists in plain sight!

Missing Out

You can see this pattern play out across so many fields, with so many talented and seemingly successful people. There are so many people who reach the absolute apex of their fields, purely by sacrificing absolutely everything else in their lives. And the sacrifice is never worth it. Sometimes, the gnawing realization that they have missed out on life can make things even worse.

It is perhaps not surprising then that people in this situation can even become suicidal. There are countless examples of people who appear superficially successful yet are dogged by demons. One such example would be the American businessman, philanthropist, film producer, and screenwriter, Steve Bing. At the age of eighteen he inherited an estimated $600 million from his grandfather. He had a high-profile career in the entertainment industry, was a major political donor, and led an often-stormy personal life. He joined "the giving pledge" set up by Bill Gates and Warren Buffet in 2012. Bing died by suicide on June 22, 2020, at the age of fifty-five by jumping from his condominium on the twenty-seventh floor of the luxury Ten Thousand building in Los Angeles. At the time of his death, his net worth was $300,000, having spent or donated most of his $600 million fortune!

In 2015, *Moneyweek* wrote about "The plight of the unhappy billionaires."[4] This article was punctuated with stories of alienation and isolation. For example, Markus Persson, the thirty-six-year-old Swedish inventor of the popular video game, Minecraft, described the immense feeling of isolation he felt after having sold his firm for $2.5 billion to Microsoft. Persson found himself "in a world every bit as isolated and purposeless as the digital one he invented." *Moneyweek* noted that his girlfriend had left him, while Persson commented, "the problem with getting everything is that you run out of reasons to keep trying. Hanging out in Ibiza with famous friends and partying with famous people, able to do whatever I want, and I've never felt more isolated."

Studies have demonstrated that, above a certain level, wealth does not equate to happiness. Naturally, it's good to be comfortable, and it's certainly preferable to be self-sufficient. Beyond that, there is no substantive evidence that becoming more successful and wealthier will lead to more happiness; in fact, if anything, becoming super-wealthy is potentially likely to lead to the opposite.

Psychologist Elizabeth Lombardo studied high-net-worth families for the book, *From Entitlement to Intention: Raising Purpose-Driven Children*. She describes in it what she terms the "treadmill effect." Lombardo notes that many people, including those who seem to be extremely successful, believe that "external things we buy will bring us happiness, but then we get them and we wonder 'what's next?' That next thing has to be bigger and better than what we had before and than what other people around us have."[5]

Not only that, but having experienced the existential emptiness associated with this realization, many financially successful people then also reflect on the immense effort they have invested in order to acquire something that has achieved absolutely nothing! Ironically, often the solution to this malady is then to sink themselves further into their work, partly in order to chase further goals that will then *finally* make them happy, and also as a deflection tactic, so they don't experience the emotional turmoil associated with actually considering the mistakes they've made in their lives. This spiral of decline can continue indefinitely, with apparently successful and highly-functioning people devolving in ever-decreasing circles, without ever addressing the actual source of their malaise.

Quite simply, their lives are tragically unbalanced. And if you asked any of these people, or indeed anyone who has achieved extraordinary wealth, they would almost certainly be willing to give up their fortune in order to experience happiness. Yet, ironically, this is often the one thing that eludes them.

It often doesn't appear that way externally. These people seem to have everything. But that can be rather misleading. The Hollywood actor Jim Carrey once tellingly said, "I think everybody should get rich and famous and do everything they ever dreamed of so they can see that it's not the answer."[6]

The Green Grass

We have all looked at someone who appears to be staggeringly successful and assumed the grass is greener on the other side of the fence. But this isn't always the case. If you imagine one of the world's most successful business people, they might have invested over eighty hours per week in their business ever since leaving school, year after year after year, possibly for decades. You may seriously be looking at an investment in the region of 200,000 hours.

In some cases, this person becomes hugely well remunerated for the effort. And so, it seems as if the pay-off is worth it. But put yourself in the shoes of this person. Would you really look back at your life with no regrets, if you invested all of your time in your career, meanwhile neglecting anything and everyone else? Almost certainly not. It is precisely this sort of person who comes to have profound regrets about the decisions they made, and they realize they have missed out on far more than they have ever accumulated. There is no level of success, no material things, no achievements, no accolades, no kudos, no praise or validation from other people that will ever compensate for that.

Yet we place these people on a pedestal. We hold them up as an example to be followed. And although they may display a particularly singular devotion, they're really not that far removed from the way many people live their lives. Many of us are treading exactly the same pathway—one of constant striving for success and achievement that is external to us. So few of us ever stop to ask the question why we behave this way.

Sacrificing for the System

Fundamentally, the individual tends to sacrifice himself or herself for the advancement of the system. That happens on both a micro and macro level; in everyday life, right up to a wider societal basis.

For example, when we consider a large organization, such as a multinational corporation, everything is ultimately geared toward achieving the best possible results for the company. The bottom line is always the bottom line. Which is ironic, as businesses invest a huge amount of time and energy in communicating precisely how interested they are in people. And, in many cases, they probably genuinely believe this and even manifest some positive signs of genuinely doing so.

But, still, ultimately businesses are set up to generate a profit for the owners and shareholders, and everything else is often extraneous, with rare exceptions. Certainly, the happiness and fulfillment of one individual worker may be completely meaningless next to the profitability of the business. It just isn't given any regard whatsoever, by comparison. This example could be extrapolated out to a variety of scenarios, but in any group situation, the ethos is almost identical. You have a pyramidal structure, with the majority of people at the bottom, and they are required to sacrifice themselves for the benefit of a tiny apex. Even people very close to the top of systems often cannot see this and are equally sacrificing their needs to achieve a goal that doesn't benefit them in the slightest.

In fact, policies, procedures, and ways of working are often implemented over such a lengthy timescale that no one can remember why they were even brought in, originally. New people who join an organization are then forced to abide by these approaches, even if it can be hugely restrictive or detrimental to their well-being. This doesn't matter; the preservation of the system is almost always what is deemed more important, rather than the needs of the individual.

This means that, aside from pursuing inauthentic goals, many people become inculcated into a way of thinking and behaving that is fundamentally unhealthy. We jettison our own desires and requirements in favor of this group orthodoxy. We become prisoners of what other people want and think, rather than express our own individuality.

We can see this reflected in so many areas of our lives. One of the primary examples must be in the insane work ethic instilled into so many of us. Surely the whole point of achieving success is so that we can afford ourselves some leisure time, the opportunity to reflect, to digest the natural world, art and culture, to spend time with our family and loved ones, and generally recharge our batteries and lead fulfilling and meaningful lives.

Cultural Programming

But this always seems to be so far down the list. Again, quite simply, this emanates from cultural programming. Particularly in the United States, there is a long-hours culture that borders on the obscene. As much as the work ethic has been lionized as a value across most countries, it is particularly strongly ingrained in the United States, where labor conditions exist that simply wouldn't be tolerated in most comparable nations. Yet, far more often than not, this is held up as some weird virtue, as if working every hour and driving yourself into an early grave is some sort of paragon of morality![7]

This is relentlessly driven home culturally, starting from our earliest days within the system. It is constantly emphasized that you must work tremendously hard in order to achieve anything, and that this should not only be your highest priority from a practical perspective, but also that it has an ethical value that even exceeds this. There is almost no greater sin than the admission that one is happy to be idle! What a strange situation—relaxation is viewed as some sort of aberration!

And the interesting thing to note is that society enabled this to happen. The technological revolution has created a situation where we can work longer hours than ever before, regardless of whether it's necessary! We were originally told that the technocracy would lead to us working less and having more hours to enjoy ourselves; think back to the news reels of the 1940s and 1950s that promoted this new manufacturing-based society of consumption. Everything was to be within our reach, and we would have all of the time in the world to enjoy it.

Endless Work

But somehow, it didn't turn out that way! In fact, the advancements of the system have perpetuated a situation in which it is possible to work almost endlessly. This simply wouldn't have been the case historically. In our primeval state, when the sun goes down, we simply go to sleep. Even just on that level alone, many people, probably the majority, are completely separated from their circadian rhythms. After all, thanks to electric lights, consumer goods, always-on broadband Internet, and many other innovations, there is no limit to the amount of time we can spend working. And, as this is actively encouraged, it's simplicity itself to get into a mindset where everything else is put on the back burner. Even sleep!

How do we deal with this lifestyle of constant striving that we have chosen? We medicate ourselves! We do things that are even worse for our health than the choices we have already made. We pump ourselves full of caffeine. We use recreational substances to anesthetize ourselves. We take prescription drugs in vast quantities. We drink and smoke to relieve stress and numb our emotional and physical pain. We destroy our bodies and minds, and in the process make the situation much worse. We become rats in an unending wheel of our own making.

It's important to emphasize at this point that we all have choices. We have to make intelligent and informed decisions about what makes sense in our lives. For example, one person may enjoy gardening or cleaning the house and gain a sense of fulfillment and achievement from doing so. That's absolutely fine. But another person may find it to be a laborious and tiring task that adds nothing to life of any value, while also piling on another layer of work to their already busy existence. In that context, it is entirely logical to hire a cleaner or gardener.

But the point is that it is not necessary to take responsibility for absolutely everything and work endlessly, believing this to be an ethical position. It makes far more sense to preserve your energy and attention for the most important tasks. Be ready to relinquish control over other aspects of your life, by delegating duties to others or working collaboratively with others who are willing to do them. Equally, if we place value in an activity, if we derive some form of worth from it, then it shouldn't be dismissed, even if it achieves no immediate monetary remuneration. And we do have an overwhelming tendency to measure value in monetary worth.

The Same Dichotomy

On one level this is logical—it comes back to the qualitative vs. quantitative dichotomy. But by doing so, we're limiting our human experience and failing to connect with the things that are actually important to us. It could be reading a book, it could be playing the piano, it could be painting, it could just be going to sleep! It could be any number of things we do not find the time to do, because we're constantly on the treadmill of working, working, working, often for someone else!!

Just before we move on!

So, in this first section of the book, we have examined why people tend to behave the ways they do, and why behaviors that are customary for large swathes of the population aren't necessarily healthy. And we've really gotten to the bottom of the socio-cultural factors that influence people's perspective and behavior.

In the next section, we're going to examine how you can recognize this in yourself, gain a greater appreciation of your identity, and set yourself on the path toward authenticity rather than imitation. This all begins with self-awareness, with a collection of different techniques and approaches that can help you move *away* from destructive and self-defeating behaviors and *toward* becoming the CEO of your life.

References

1. Gillett, R. (2015). "From welfare to one of the world's wealthiest women — the incredible rags-to-riches story of J.K. Rowling." *Business Insider.*

2. Menin, A. (2022). "From Bill Gates to Mark Zuckerberg: the college drop-outs who built a fortune." *The Times.*

3. Wong, K., Chan, A. & Ngan, S. (2019). "The Effect of Long Working Hours and Overtime on Occupational Health: A Meta-Analysis of Evidence from 1998 to 2018." *International Journal of Environmental Research and Public Research.* June 2019. Issue 16, Vol. 12: 2102.

4. *Moneyweek.* (2015). "The Plight of the Unhappy Billionaires."

5. Kirsten, L. Aurora, S. & Thomas, T. (2021). "Are the Rich Actually Wealthy?" *DayCreekHowl.*

6. Kim, L. (2015). "I Think Everyone Should Get Rich and Famous: What Did Jim Carrey Actually Mean?" *Medium.*

7. Abadi, M. (2017). "6 American work habits people in other countries think are ridiculous." *The Independent.*

NOTES

_____

_____

_____

_____

_____

_____

_____

_____

_____

_____

_____

_____

_____

_____

_____

_____

_____

_____

_____

_____

_____

_____

_____

_____

_____

_____

_____

_____

_____

_____

_____

_____

PART II

INNER EXCELLENCE

Chapter 4

Be Aware

IN THE FIRST PART of this book, we established that many people lead a self-limited existence and do not realize their true potential. Virtually everyone tends to believe that their desires and goals are almost entirely self-directed. Yet, in reality, there are a multitude of factors that actually influence what we deem to be important and the various choices we make or think we make, as discussed in the limited-self model. And it is often impossible to decipher this process, if we don't develop awareness.

In this chapter, we will begin to explore a timeless "Awareness" model that we developed. You can apply this immediately to all areas of your life, make huge shifts, move the needle, and start seeing results almost right away. Moreover, also enjoy the ride!

Inside not Outside

You have the solution inside you. You do not have to seek an external solution. You don't have to get a PhD in neuroscience. You don't have to master ancient scriptures and textbooks. You don't need to become a psychologist. You don't need to make a billion dollars; in fact, you don't even have to spend or invest large amounts of money! You don't have to fill your life with striving and craving. If you begin the journey to lasting happiness with inner fulfillment and inner excellence, this will then naturally manifest as happiness in the world you experience externally.

Somehow, we have been tricked into looking outside ourselves for contentment. This is perhaps not surprising; we live in such a capitalistic, commercialized, and media-driven world, this inevitably impacts on our perspective. What we believe to be our own desires in the marketplace are often primarily influenced by external factors rather than true desire, and this is supported by academic research.

But this artificial bubble can be burst so easily, once we develop awareness. The value of self-awareness is that it allows us to develop the thoughts, emotions, and patterns of behavior that are supportive of our authentic needs and desires, rather than running contrary to them. And this awareness is not something obscure, remote, or untouchable. Attaining it doesn't require you to spend decades in a Tibetan retreat. You don't need to become an expert at tantric yoga. It's achievable in the here and now, via very simple techniques that people can begin to implement today. The more you focus on your awareness, the more it will come to the forefront of your life, and the more you will then be directed by who you really are. This can only be a massive positive.

On the next page, see the Awareness Model:

The Awareness Model

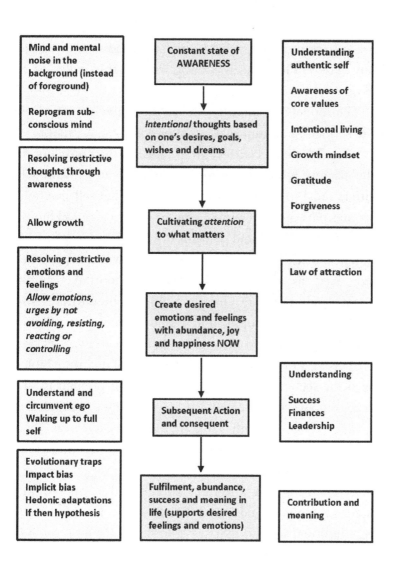

In order to address this notion of awareness, we would firstly like to introduce this model of awareness we have developed. Through the remainder of this book, we will discuss various aspects of this model and how to apply them immediately. Please keep coming back to this image as you see fit.

The model is primarily focused on achieving what could be described as an improved state of consciousness, of being, of "I Am." It begins with reprogramming the conscious and subconscious mind so that attention is cultivated toward what matters most to the individual. The more that self-awareness becomes part of our reality, the more we can let go of limiting thoughts, emotions, and patterns of behavior.

For centuries and across the globe, awareness has been recognized as a core principle. Its importance is well documented in ancient literature, modern literature, Eastern and Western philosophy and wisdom, doctrinal religions, spirituality, yoga, and mysticism, to name a few. Such is its impact that now, a modern scientific field of quantum biology has been recognized and is gaining wide popularity. The concept of awareness explains that we are not our mind, brain (intellect), or body. Rather, we are the "consciousness" that is aware of our mind, body, thoughts, feelings, and behavior/actions.

By focusing our attention and intention on our most important authentic desires and goals, we create the thoughts and emotional state(s) that are desirable. This then produces an abundance mindset and belief system that enables us to take appropriate (and massive) action in our lives. As we understand our authentic selves and core values, a new mode of intentional living surfaces, and the sort of social, financial, and lifestyle success we truly desire in order to be happy becomes part of our experience.

Overarching the whole concept of the "awareness model" is the idea of "creating a constant state of awareness." This might sound like a daunting prospect, but it is actually predicated on some relatively simple processes. In order to become constantly aware, it's important to start actively behaving in an aware fashion, conducting some straightforward exercises, some of which are described below. If you're able to follow through on this commitment, your whole state of perception and being will begin to evolve.

Core Values

A great place to start with the whole process of self-awareness is to establish your core values.

Now, most people probably believe they already know their core values. But often, they have been steered in the wrong direction by external forces. There is a psychological phenomenon, referred to as the Barnum-Forer effect, whereby some people are inclined to give credence to descriptions of themselves and their lives that are broadly applicable to many people.[1] So, for example, they might believe that a horoscope has figured everything out, without the need for any investment of time in self-knowledge. Everything is laid out for them, so they therefore don't have to actually bother to know anything about themselves!

Thus, establishing your own authentic core values is key. And there are many tests and exercises available that will enable you to explore this important topic (see author note at the end of the chapter). There is no better place to begin with the journey of self-discovery, because these core values represent the things that are most important to you, whether you are aware of them or not.

So, if your core value is compassion, you will always automatically gravitate toward compassion in your life choices. You should find a field where you can really help other people, as you will simply find this more edifying. Of course, the majority of people will gain some sense of purpose from this process, but many are not actually driven by compassion as such. In a caring profession, for example, they may enjoy aspects of the job but experience frustration at other elements. The same may also apply to people who have compassion at their core, but they will never feel unfulfilled or defeated by these frustrations, as this quality of compassion is their driving force, their raison d'être.

The Core of Your Existence

Once you have established these core values, whatever they might be (and there are no right or wrong answers!), you can then begin the process of bringing these qualities into the core of your existence. This can be a difficult step, as people often wonder how they can place compassion, empathy, freedom, security, loyalty, or other personal qualities at the center of their lives.

Fundamentally, your core values need to make the journey from your subconscious mind to your everyday reality. You want always to be aware of them; they are central to your daily existence. This simply requires you to develop a new state of awareness, one in which you cultivate attention to the things that really matter to you.

There are a variety of ways to achieve this; implementing as many of them as possible is certainly advisable.

A great way to begin is to make your core values visible in your life. Write them down, for example on a Post-it Note, and then place them near where you work or where you spend the majority of your time. This doesn't have to be a deep or extensive document. It can simply be several short phrases that encompass the most important things to your soul and being. The important thing is to keep them on hand, ensuring they're always conscious in your brain as you go about your day. This will mean you don't have to dig into your subconscious to bring them to mind.

People and Values

Opening the channels of communication with people who are close to you on the subject is also valuable. Why not discuss your core values with close family and friends?

This has two benefits. First, simply by having conversations with peers, you are bringing these important concepts into your conscious awareness, meaning you are less likely to be ruled by your subconscious; ergo, the more your core values seep into your conscious awareness, the more you're going to act on them. And second, these people who are close to you can help hold you to account. If they understand your core values, they understand you better as a person and can help nudge you in the right direction, if they see you going awry. Having such frank and insightful discussions with friends and family can even strengthen your relationships with them.

In accordance with this, you might even find that you need to tweak the people who are in your life. It's not always the case that the people who are closest to us are positive inputs. There are many negative people in the world, and while these people will hopefully get on the right track someday, it's nonetheless often necessary to eliminate those who do not resonate with our values and beliefs, in order to ensure we are surrounding ourselves with positivity.

People that are close to you do not need to share your beliefs—we are all different, after all. But they do need to be supportive of who you are and not play a role in steering you away from positive and constructive behaviors.

Self-Assessment and Cultivation

Another practical step you can take to be in alignment with your core values is to go through a process every morning of assessing your day and what you have to achieve.

List the tasks you intend to accomplish, and then assess whether they are commensurate with your core values. If you find yourself doing lots of things that don't mesh with the person you are, it's time to reassess your life. If you're continually doing things that run contrary to your core values, then, no matter how productive you might appear, you will never end up being fulfilled. If you complete the exercise several times and find that, on most days, you are doing things that are not consistent with your deep-rooted inner values, then it's time to reflect on how you can change your life to achieve this.

This process can also be supplemented by integrating your core values into everyday conversations. The people who tend to be the happiest and live the most liberated lives are those who voice their inner values regularly. If you make your core values part of your everyday lexicon of language, then it naturally follows that you'll remember them and bring them to mind more readily. This will then positively impact on your behavior and outlook, creating a virtuous circle.

Just as you begin your day by putting your core values at the center of everything you do, you should also end your day that way as well. Evaluate every day at bedtime, and assess whether you have managed to stay consistent with your core values. If there is room for improvement, then you can address that the next day.

This is valuable generally, as it also moors you in the present. Instead of just directing your attention toward some future or imagined goal, focusing on making every day as good as it can possibly be and in accordance with your core values is a much more effective way to have an enjoyable and fulfilling life.

If you follow this pattern every day, it will become habit-forming, and suddenly bringing your core values into your conscious awareness will be less necessary.

The Power of Now

This life philosophy has been conveyed memorably in the work of Eckhart Tolle, particularly his seminal work, *The Power of Now*. This book asserts that only the present moment is real and only the present moment matters. Both the past and the future are manufactured by our minds. We imagine a future that may never come, and we dwell on a past that doesn't matter in this moment.[2]

Tolle suggests a range of relaxation and meditational methods in order to reprogram behavior and anchor oneself in the present. These suggestions include slowing down by avoiding multitasking, spending time in nature, and letting go of worries about the future. Acceptance of "what is" without judgment of good or bad, desirable or undesirable, or any such other duality is a primal step.[3] Definitely food for thought and an important contribution to becoming closer to who we truly are.

Once you have instigated this basic process of living in a way that is consistent with your core values, you can begin to approach the concept on a broader scale. Your personal core values in the state of awareness should inform every major decision you make, and arguably every minor decision you make, as well! But certainly, major life events should be viewed through the lens of who you really are.

Every opportunity, goal, or decision can be seen as a chance to create harmony in your existence rather than conflict. Take a couple of days every few months to engage in strategic planning. Assess the direction of your life, and consider whether your objectives and core values mesh effectively. When your mind, body, values, and everyday life are all in sync, great things begin to happen.

Visualizing and Living your Ideal

As greater awareness of your true self increasingly seeps into your consciousness, there are a variety of other things you can do in order to accelerate and cement this process

First, visualizing your ideal self can be extremely valuable. We all have an image in our minds of who we'd like to be. Exploring this can be a critical step on the path to self-knowledge, as often we will find that there is a chasm between who we are and who we want to be. If this is the case, try jotting down some practical steps that will help you move closer to your ideal self.

Ultimately, what we actually *do* is central to living an actualized existence. So, putting activities at the forefront of your conscious transition to your ideal self is vital. This can work on two levels. First, determining what you're passionate about and then pursuing your passions is logical and powerful. Vast numbers of people want to spend their lives doing things they're passionate about, but so few people manage to do it. Instead of playing it safe, consider what really matters to you and excites you. Identifying this is the first step to filling your life with it.

Additionally, experimenting with new activities can be highly constructive. How can you know if something will inspire you, if you've never tried it?! The more new activities you attempt, the more you will learn about yourself. This is valuable information that can really help steer you in the right direction in life, as you gain insight into the things that make you tick as a human being.

Many people also go through their lives without properly assessing their skillsets. It's natural for us to enjoy things more when we're good at them. Yet many of us often don't consider our skills too closely; instead, we plow on in an existing job because it pays well. Sitting down and thinking about your skillset can be a critical component of self-knowledge and a great way to identify new opportunities for yourself. This can help steer you in an unexpected but inspiring new direction.

Unconscious Direction

It is surprising how often people's lives are akin to a beach ball on the ocean, bobbing around unconsciously, being pushed and pulled by forces over which they have no control, unable to stop and assess why they are in the ocean in the first place!

To give you an example of this, one friend of ours was the only child of immigrant parents, who had emigrated to the United States from South Korea. It has been instilled in this person from an early age that his parents had worked from 6 a.m. to 8 p.m., seven days a week, just to provide for their children. This message was hammered home repeatedly, not for any malignant or malicious reasons, but simply because the parents believed that this hard work had been fundamental to their existence. Without that drive, they would never have made it in America.

This then reflected on the attitude of this person, as his perspective was inevitably influenced by his parents, particularly as they drilled this message home relentlessly during his formative years. Inevitably, instead of questioning what role he wished to fulfill in society or attempting to work out how he wanted his life to look in the future, he ended up following the wishes and desires of his parents. So, he went down the frequent route for Asian children of studying extremely hard and working toward medical qualifications.

But, at a certain point during his existence, this person questioned why he had actually attended medical school. He had been getting into Myers-Briggs and some other psychological indicators at the time, and this had led him to question his entire existence. And when he reflected on the medical school question, he couldn't actually conceive of a satisfactory answer. He acknowledged that the default answer would be that he enjoyed science, which was true, but ultimately, the most prevailing fact was simply that his parents had wanted him to attend medical school.

The more he considered this issue, the more he realized he had taken the path of least resistance, and that his course through life barely reflected his own preferences. Again, when he picked a residency within medicine, he had chosen family medicine. Upon reflection, the reason for this was that it was the path of least resistance and required the least mental effort in order to pursue it.

Your career is one side of the life coin. The other is what you wish to achieve and experience outside of your work. This same person reflected that his life goals were to be financially successful, married with children, and generally leading a healthy life. This would obviously be a common set of objectives, yet somehow this person believed it was a vague and perhaps inauthentic picture. He felt that the desires were not really his own; the goals were certainly not ones he truly understood and were more reflective of his cultural background than personal passion.

In fact, he had little concept of what being married would be like or, indeed, how much money he needed to live comfortably. These were intangibles that he was seeking, rather than his own tangible goals. Indeed, he would never have known if he'd actually reached his goals, since they had never been properly defined. This led to a deep period of self-reflection, during which he studied self-awareness and realized that *this* would define his existence going forward. This was the *aha! moment.*

Constructive Exercises and Emotional Intelligence

This is where there are numerous exercises that can assist you with examining your identity and understanding your core beliefs and personality. Myers-Briggs Type Indicator and the Enneagram of Personality models and assessments can assist in steering someone in the right direction.

Many people effectively sleepwalk through their lives. To quote Oscar Wilde, "Most people are other people. Their thoughts are someone else's opinions, their lives a mimicry, their passions a quotation."[4] That was a rather acerbic observation, but the point remains that, as in the example just given, many people go through life simply fulfilling the roles that have been set out for them, without ever questioning it, getting to know themselves properly, or working out how their lives could be happier and more successful on their terms.

In particular, understanding and developing your emotional intelligence, often described as EQ, can be particularly useful. Most people are fully conversant with the concept of IQ, yet it is EQ that can often be the path to a successful life.

Psychologists Michael Beldoch and Daniel Goleman were instrumental in the development of this important aspect of human understanding,[5] and it has become increasingly advocated by the mental health and business communities as a vital quality of high-functioning people.

Fundamentally, emotional intelligence represents the ability to understand, use, and manage emotions in positive ways to relieve stress, communicate effectively, empathize with others, overcome challenges, and defuse conflict. It is defined by self-management, self-awareness, social awareness, and relationship management. Studies indicate that EQ is a much more accurate indicator of success and happiness than IQ,[6] which means it is something we should all work toward developing.

So much of emotional intelligence is related to awareness. It takes its cue from the ability to recognize emotions in yourself and others, which is really at the core of the awareness model. Self-awareness is about moving from a situation where you do things on autopilot and don't know why, to doing things consciously, in awareness of your core values, regularly assessing the direction you're headed in and how you can align this better with your authentic self.

Emotional intelligence impacts on every aspect of your life: your performance in work or education; your mental health; your physical well-being; as well as your personal relationships. And you can build this quality at any time, simply by considering its constituent parts and taking action to develop those characteristics within yourself.

Managing Emotions

Central to emotional intelligence is the management of emotions. The way people experience and deal with emotions can vary greatly, and this can have a profound impact on the way their lives turn out.

Being aware of your emotions is a key aspect of emotional intelligence, something that can slip under the radar. Many people are not aware of the degree to which they inhibit or repress their emotions, so addressing this can be a critical pillar of developing true self-awareness.

The best way to identify this is to address the following questions:

- ❖ Do you experience emotions that vary rapidly?
- ❖ When you are emotional, do you experience physical sensations in your stomach, throat, or chest?
- ❖ Do you experience individual feelings and emotions, such as anger, sadness, fear, and joy, each of which is evident in subtle facial expressions?

❖ Do you experience intense feelings that capture your attention?

❖ Do your emotions play a major role in your decision-making?

If these experiences are unfamiliar, it strongly suggests you may be dimming down or turning off your emotions.

One of the best ways to reconnect with your emotions is through a practice of mindfulness: the basic human ability to be fully present, aware of where you are and what you're doing. The cultivation of mindfulness has roots in Buddhism, and mindfulness practice requires you to purposely focus your attention on the present moment. This can be a key tool in the goal of developing emotional, social, and self-awareness. From this point, your ability to manage challenging situations, express and deal with your own emotional states, and connect with your own authentic self will all increase.

Speaking with a therapist or a coach can also be part of this process of self-discovery. Exploring issues and looking within yourself for answers can be hugely beneficial.

Regardless of what matters to you, it is only by understanding and claiming this uniqueness and authenticity that you can achieve leadership in your own life. There is no one less free in this world than someone in a prison of their own making, who can't even see the bars they have created.

Influential Thinkers

The ideas discussed in this chapter have been espoused by many influential thinkers, writers, and researchers. Dr. Joe

Dispenza is one such academic; he has brought attention to the topic of self-awareness and how important it is to master the thoughts that control our personal habits.

Dispenza asserts that most people begin their days by thinking about their problems, and these issues tend to be attached to people, places, and situations with emotional connotations.[7] This is why breaking this chain and focusing on your authentic self and core values from the start of the day can be such a powerful technique; it breaks the negative bonds that restrict many people's lives. Dispenza asserts that by following this tendency, people become trapped in their biology. An emotional state is created that ensnares people, and this inevitably leads to a situation where people are living in the past. This then prevents them from taking positive action in the present.

There are similarities here with the teachings of Dr. Gabor Maté, considered an expert in the fields of trauma, addiction, stress, and childhood development. Maté asserts that most addiction emanates from relationships with emotional trauma based in the past. Only by bringing this emotion into a state of awareness and addressing it can the pattern of addiction be broken. [8]

Really, what both of these researchers are talking about is the difference between mind and awareness. Many people live in a state of mind and believe it to be a state of awareness. But it's certainly not a state of self-awareness; it is often merely a system of conditioned responses.

Evolving beyond this is critical in an environment that can often be hostile to self-awareness, precisely because it requires you to be trapped in an unending state of desire, striving, and goal-seeking, so you will be an ideal consumer.

Summary

There are two primary takeaways from this chapter.

First, developing awareness of yourself and bringing this into the forefront of your life is critically important, if you wish to lead a happy and fulfilled existence.

Second, there are simple yet concrete exercises you can conduct to develop this self-awareness. This means that self-awareness and, ultimately, success, fulfillment, and happiness are not the exalted or elusive goal we might believe.

Start practicing now!

Multiple times a day, notice "*awareness.*" Don't change anything, just notice! Even if nothing happens, don't rush. Keep noticing.

Notice that you are not your body or mind. You are the consciousness that is *aware* of your mind, brain, and body.

Notice the space around you. Don't attach labels or opinions. Just notice.

Just be. Don't judge. Let your awareness grow.

Notice yourself, how you feel inside. What does your body feel like?

Notice your self-talk, your thoughts, your emotions, your reactions. Notice your habits. Notice your actions. Notice your interactions.

Don't force any thoughts or emotions or expect to feel anything. Let it come naturally. Become aware, and let it fill your entire consciousness. Slowly, you will feel an expanding aura of consciousness.

Before you do something, try to bring consciousness into it. Are you doing this in a state of awareness? Notice. Take a few seconds.

Awareness is within reach of everyone. We are our conscious awareness!

Practice consistently!

Further Work and Reading

We authors have developed and now conduct an exclusive mastermind workshop to accurately identify, define and map your personal core values.

Contact us at legendaryquestpro@gmail.com for more information.

References

1. *Encyclopedia Britannica.* (2022). "Barnum Effect."

2. Göke, N. (2020). "Eckhart Tolle's Way of Looking at Time Will Make You Happier Today." *Medium.*

3. Saviuc, L. (2022). Eckhart Tolle Speaks on Acceptance and Surrender. PurposeFairy.

4. Oxford Reference. (2022). *Oscar Wilde 1854–1900 Irish dramatist and poet - Quotations.*

5. *Learning in Action.* (2018). "What is Emotional Intelligence? And What's Missing?"

6. Cotruş, A., Stanciu, C., & Bulborea, A. (2012). "EQ vs. IQ Which is Most Important in the Success or Failure of a Student?" *Procedia - Social and Behavioral Sciences*, Volume 46, 2012, pp. 5211-5213

7. *The Indian Express*. (2020). "Don't wait for tragedy, you can also change your life in a state of joy and inspiration."

8. Moorhead, J. (2018). "How dealing with past trauma may be the key to breaking addiction." *The Guardian*.

NOTES

_____

_____

_____

_____

_____

_____

_____

_____

_____

_____

_____

_____

_____

_____

_____

_____

Chapter 5

Thoughts and Feelings are Optional

HUMAN BEINGS ARE full of thoughts and emotions. There is no getting away from that. This is undoubtedly part of the human experience. We're not here in this chapter or book to condemn thoughts or emotions or feeling emotional. But it's also important to recognize and understand that our thoughts and emotions are *not* the totality of who we are, and they shouldn't dictate our outlook or behavior. Moreover, any thoughts or emotions are optional. This often comes as a total shock for many people!

Thinking the Thoughts

Every single one of us has more than fifty thousand thoughts each day. Most people believe these thoughts are random and just happen to appear in their mindscape based on their past, present, or future (desires) (see limited-self model); essentially, based on a range of parameters as discussed in the introductory part of this book. Repeated thoughts (combined with emotions and perceptions) become our beliefs, our preferences or prejudices, our belief system, our very own version of truth. So, do we have a choice?

What if, instead, you were able to choose your own thoughts? What if you were the conscious awareness that was watching your thoughts and deciding which thoughts should be predominant? This doesn't mean controlling or resisting your thoughts; rather, it means choosing which you will focus on and which you will relinquish.

This is also not about judging your thoughts. It's about letting go non-judgmentally of any thoughts you don't wish to focus on. Truly speaking our thoughts leads to further emotions, which can lead to more thoughts. Together, this process fuels our behavior patterns and actions.

Our subconscious or deep patterns will often instinctively direct thoughts and emotions, especially during stressful situations or whenever we encounter perceived threats. This is another reason many people think they have no choice over their thoughts and emotions. However, this is simply not true.

As we start focusing our attention intentionally on the thoughts we desire, while letting go of others that are undesirable, we slowly begin reprogramming our conscious and subconscious mind. Over time, with consistent practice, our subconscious mind can be completely recalibrated, and no matter how deep-rooted the thoughts and beliefs have been, they can be shifted. And, thus, our emotional experience and reality will undergo a similar process of positive transformation.

Responding Emotionally

Emotions are a certain type(s) of vibration(s) in your body, often with a physical adjunct. This is distinct from sensations such as pain, which is the psychical adjunct of an imperative protective reflex.

For example, when we lash out at others in condemnation, this is an emotional response. Deep down, we know this, despite how much we attempt to convince ourselves that we are responding rationally or in accordance with our values. This may also be true, but it isn't what drives the behavior. It has an emotional foundation. This has actually become a cultural trope within our society, with profound division often evident between polemical factions. Tolerance for opposing views or contrasting behavior seems to be on the wane. Again, this is often based on emotion rather than reason. We all recognize that freedom of speech and expression are important, yet it has become increasingly common to attempt to silence what we perceive to be dissenting voices.

We repeat: emotions are part of us but not who we are. This can be easily proven. Have you ever responded strongly to something, clearly in an emotional fashion, and then, at a later date, possibly within a matter of minutes, regretted your conduct? Hands up, everyone who has experienced that! We would expect to see everyone's hands at this point!

There are biological reasons for our having emotions, and they can serve a purpose. Emotional states are a mechanism of defense and protection. But they can also hamstring us and cause us to behave in a way that is detrimental to our well-being, as well as to other people's.

So, what we need to do is learn to observe our emotions and even to observe other people's emotional states. Become a master of observation! This is a non-judgmental and non-attached approach to life, to yourself and to others, one that serves the totality of who you are as a fully-formed being.

Taking Ownership

The first part of the process is to take ownership of your own conduct. And this begins with being an active observer of your own behavior, thoughts, and, particularly, emotions. When we lash out at others, this is always an emotional reaction. It's not rational; it's not based on a cost-benefit analysis, as we rarely benefit! And it's certainly not coming from the heart, from a place of empathy, from a place of love and oneness.

This applies to so many of our thoughts, so many of our feelings. They are very often programmed reactions. They are not rational impulses. In fact, if you examine many of your attitudes to life, whether referring to your life or other people's, you will almost inevitably reflect that they are not based on a rational assessment of the situation but rather on an often-deep-seated emotion.

This is why learning to observe your own emotions and thought processes is so important. When you notice yourself complaining, moaning, judging, acting hatefully, being vengeful, or exhibiting other negative patterns of behavior, both toward yourself and others, watch yourself and stop yourself gently! If anything, you are compromising your own chances of success and fulfillment, since this negativity then becomes the predominant emotion prevailing in your consciousness.

Behavior begins with thoughts, so become a master of your own mind. When you slide into a negative mindset in which these self-sabotaging responses emerge, correct yourself. Create a positive internal dialogue from a space of acceptance, non-judgment, and abundance. Make this a habit. It will soon become a virtuous circle, and then second nature.

When we react strongly to some petty incident—it could be on social media, it could be unnecessary road rage, it could be snapping at someone when we feel aggrieved at work, and particularly when we're piqued by someone else having the temerity to hold an opposing viewpoint to our own(!)—what we're actually doing is projecting. We're projecting our own insecurities, our own inadequacies, our own discomfort with our state of self, and then using that internalized dissatisfaction as the fuel to lash out at someone else. It is seldom anything to do with the other person. It virtually always comes from within, as do all of our impulses and emotional reactions.

Negative Self-Talk

That negative self-talk that you torture yourself with... Hardly rational, is it? It comes from thoughts and emotions, it comes from learned behavior, it comes from negative tendencies we create within our own minds and nervous systems. We even cement these processes by changing our mind maps and neuronal structure permanently, meaning we continue with the same self-defeating spiral of negative thoughts, negative emotions, negative behaviors, and negative outcomes.

So, here is something of substance to take away right now. Whenever you're tempted to launch a stinging riposte at someone, whenever you feel like angrily beeping your horn at another road user, whenever you're about to deliver a withering put-down on Twitter, whenever you're berating yourself over some trivial incident... pause, observe the process, observe the way you feel internally. And realize it's not about them, it's not about the social poster, the inept motorist, or the outspoken polemicist. It's all about you. It's all about the way you feel about yourself. And when you stop feeling this way, when you're happy with who you are, when you respect yourself, when you radiate love, empathy, and happiness, you won't have the remotest interest in behaving that way any longer.

We are certainly not advising that you accept or tolerate any form of abuse or physical harm. Healthy boundaries are certainly necessary! We are talking about taking total responsibility for your own emotions without blaming anyone (including yourself).

In addition to your own emotions, learn to become a keen observer of everything and everyone you see around you. Constantly remind yourself that everyone else is just like you. And when someone does or says something that begins to attract your ire, take a step back, check yourself, and remember that he or she is an autonomous human being as well. If they have expressed themselves in a way you disagree with, respect their right to a different viewpoint and perspective.

If they have, for example, bumped into you in a supermarket or cut in front of you at a traffic light, don't fly off the handle. Don't instantly assume this is a malicious, thoughtless, selfish monster! This person is human. They have good moments, bad moments, strong qualities, human failings, up days, and down days, as we all do. Accept people as they are and the world as it is, not as you wish them to be. Celebrate and accept the human, rather than repress and suppress it.

And never forget that, while we are often slaves to certain restrictive and febrile emotions, this rarely, if ever, results in constructive outcomes. We might feel we really need to respond to certain things, but if nothing good comes of these responses, then how does this serve us, as people?

Emotional not Intellectual

And such reactions are emotional, no matter how much we are convinced of the intellectual rightness of our views, because the intellect would tell us that sniping at other people, belittling the arguments of others, attacking opposing viewpoints, creating arguments and conflict, and entering into negative cycles of self-defeating behavior never ends positively. It never makes us feel good! It never achieves anything! We never acquire anything of substance from the process; in fact, we usually end up feeling bad!

As you begin to watch how people express themselves and bring this issue into your consciousness, you will gather a new corpus of knowledge that will enable you to expand yourself as a social agent. You have vast potential, with the ability to develop new proteins and latent software. But these will only be activated when you are challenged in new ways. And if you challenge yourself to see people in the context of love (unconditional love) or try to identify win-win situations or endeavor to make smart decisions on behalf of yourself and others, these new modes and methods of thinking will strengthen over time. Slowly but surely, you will evolve into a new being.

Psychologists and those who study human behavior sometimes describe a similar process as *metacognition*, the ability to reflect and critically analyze how you think. An academic paper published in China in 2019 deeply examined the role of metacognition in several areas of our lives. It concluded that metacognition can have a positive role in numerous areas, particularly in fostering creativity and creative thinking.[1] This is precisely the area we wish to address in this chapter: cultivating positive, constructive, creative thoughts and emotions, instead of negative, reductive, restrictive processes.

If we can take a step back, make a mental count to ten, allow our emotions to cool down to simmering from boiling over like an overheated saucepan, and then finally reach a temperate level, we will experience much more empathy with others. This then becomes a habit and heightens our mindset, mentality, and state of being, while opening up our hearts and minds.

Tolle's Internal Landscape

Another important aspect of this tendency to criticize has been discussed by the spiritual teacher and best-selling author Eckhart Tolle. His concept of the pain-body provides a fascinating insight into how unreasonable we are being when we ask others to change their views for little reason other than to satisfy our own egos.[2]

Tolle notes that the internal landscape of every person is vast, complex, and highly individual. That applies to every single one of us. Who could possibly understand your inner workings or the myriad factors and the interplay between them that has resulted in your personality and beliefs today? Even you would struggle to fully understand it, so what chance has anyone else of understanding?

The same applies equally when you observe someone else. You don't know what this person has been through, what they have experienced, what knowledge they have acquired, and all manner of other components of their existence that have contributed to their overall psychology, mentality, and worldview. They could have been through horrifying trauma, they may have been rejected horribly and feel fundamentally unloved, they might have lived in a warzone; in fact, any number of interpersonal and family relationships may impact on their sense of self and viewpoint.

You have absolutely no chance of ever truly understanding everything they've been through, even if they explain every last morsel of their life experience to you! Instead, you should seek to empathize with them. You should seek to acknowledge the fact that they have a right to their opinion and that their opinion has the same validity as yours. You should not seek to chastise, correct, or conquer them. You should love and respect them and intrinsically understand that imposing your ideas on others means effectively asking them to rearrange their internal landscape for your benefit. Why on Earth should they do this? Would you do the same for them? What you're doing is akin to inviting yourself into their home and then rearranging all of their furniture without invitation. You wouldn't do that. So don't try to rearrange their mental, emotional, and psychic furniture!

Thus, taking full responsibility for your own thoughts, emotions, and behavior is your golden armor, whilst letting others do the same. This is among the surest way to fulfillment. As the ancient scriptures describe it, gain control over your mind rather than let it control you! Tame the tigers within, not those outside!

Ingroups and Outgroups

We are increasingly encouraged to see ourselves as part of an in-group and then collectively vilify an out-group. These terms were popularized by the Polish social psychologist Henri Tajfel;[3] they have rarely been more apt than in our contemporary society.

The mainstream media chisels away at our sense of self, until we identify with a group more than our real self. That's why a big part of waking up to ourselves, in our opinion, is about taking time to disconnect from mass media, breaking our screen addiction, and decoupling ourselves from the toxic messages it continually pumps out (which also, ironically, claim to be against toxic behavior!).

We are not White, Black, female, male, American, British, European, African, working-class, middle-class, poor, rich, old, young, gay, straight, Republican, Democrat, right-wing, left-wing, or any other divisive label. This is not how we should identify ourselves, and we definitely shouldn't demonize those who don't share our particular affiliations. We are human beings and are our own conscious awareness. We are not defined by our differences but instead by our similarities. And we won't live life to the fullest or realize the true potential of society until we permanently wake up to this reality.

Mindfulness Practice

A practice that can assist with this transformation is *mindfulness*, defined as being fully present and aware of where we are and what we're doing. Bringing your focus to the present moment enables you to just be, to connect with the higher level of your essential self.

Guided meditation and yoga can assist with this process, helping to center you in the present moment and further cultivating the mind-body connection. Kundalini yoga is particularly valuable, as it plays an active role in awakening and healing the energy body, along with releasing trauma blocks. Mindfulness meditation also helps to cultivate a sense of awareness in the individual, teaching us to look inward, observe our experience, and learn to let go. *Autobiography of a Yogi* by Paramahansa Yogananda is a seminal text that introduces people to this area.

This is all very much part of the process of connecting with the heart and the spirit. But we can't complete this process until we've removed all of the blockages. And part of this process is accepting and rewriting our personal story. As discussed in the previous chapter, many people have been running from their pain for a long time. Ironically, when we fail to address this critical constituent of our makeup, we don't eliminate pain from our existence; instead, pain becomes our story.

Observing Others

Another aspect of observation is observing others. When you look around on a daily basis, whether in the offline or online world, observe the habits of other people. The way they behave. The way they treat others. Ask yourself whether you want to be akin to the worst examples you witness, which may be many!

Do you want to treat people as objects to be used? Do you want to trample all over people? Do you want to be rude and dismissive? Do you want to treat life as an unending competition and quest for supremacy? Do you want to lose your temper frequently and lash out angrily at the slightest incident? Is that the path to enlightenment, fulfillment, happiness, and a healthy society and self?

When you place yourself and others under the microscope, almost inevitably you will conclude that there is much you could, would, and should change. How often have you found your mood turning on a dime over the most trivial things? This is surprisingly common. But it's something we should all strive to overcome, as it does us a disservice. It's a jarring process that disconnects us from our true selves.

And the interesting and important thing to note about it is that we create this! This shift in mood and mentality is not caused by the event itself. It's caused by our reaction to it. We tend to think of emotions arising because of an event, and certainly these can be the trigger for the emotions. But we create an emotional mood by our own insistence that we must cling to this emotion, keeping it alive with our thought processes.

We replay events over and over in our minds, and eventually our mood is lowered. Sometimes, we even delve further into the issue than it deserves, attributing some deeper meaning to an innocuous occurrence. *Is this what everyone else thinks about me? Am I not good enough?* And so on. This one incident, that may have lasted mere seconds, can even trigger responses that last for years.

To give an extreme example, in the British media recently, there has been a notable case of stalking that involves the broadcaster, Emily Maitlis. A gentleman whom she met at Cambridge University has been pestering her for over thirty years. He has completely ruined his life and is currently serving a prison sentence in relation to this stalking. Yet still, despite being in this situation, despite having been told by a judge that he has destroyed his own life and made Ms. Maitlis's quite miserable at times, it has been reported that he is still writing to her, wanting apparent closure on some minor incident that occurred in 1990![4]

This is a classic—albeit rare, given its intensity and moral dubiousness—example of allowing an emotion connected with an event to fester and grow out of all proportion. When we allow this to happen, we disenfranchise ourselves from the higher self, from the side of us that can achieve success, harmony, and bliss; instead, we become consumed with a negative mindset. We foster a mentality that is disconnected, disengaged, and decoupled from others, from the infinite universe, and from who we really are.

Physical Place

Whenever we experience these sensations, we should remind ourselves that they are just a vibration in our body. Any emotion is felt as a vibration! Yet, because of our analytical minds, we over-analyze the emotion. We ask ourselves why we feel a certain way, when the reality is that our physical bodies have prompted and manifested this sensation.

It is these answers, this process of cogitation, that perpetuates and prolongs what should be a transitory emotion. The considering, contemplating, ruminating, and questioning we all go through dramatically extends the lifecycle of what often should be fleeting sensations. And, even more crucially, the experience becomes incorrectly interpreted. We become one with our emotions, identify with them, and even drown in them. The negativity spirals out of control!

That's why it's so important to remind ourselves that we are the consciousness experiencing the physical sensations and emotional responses in our body. This will make it so much easier to be an observer. You can almost watch the emotion arise, noticing that the emotional feeling can disappear, even if the physical discomfort persists.

When emotions arise, go straight into your head, and ask yourself what you're thinking and what is triggering these responses. Record the sensations you feel in your body. Note them down on paper. That way, you will recognize them and be ready to deal with them, the next time you encounter them. Do not try to control, resist, or avoid the emotions. Let them be!

Cultivating Thoughts and Emotions

Cultivating the emotions and thoughts we actually want to feel is critically important. We cannot control our thoughts and, particularly, our feelings, but we can choose them. We can decide which feelings and thoughts we allow to take root, and we can also encourage positive thoughts and emotions to perpetuate by creating constructive processes.

Breathing exercises can help in this process. Center yourself in the present with slow, deep breaths. Allow yourself to relax. Imagine yourself in a safe and peaceful place. Remind yourself that you are neither your emotions nor your thoughts. You are, instead, the observer, creator, and choice-maker of your emotions and thoughts. Celebrate this! You are always in charge of your internal processes, regardless of the situation and circumstances.

Accept your feelings. Allow yourself to be confident that you can handle the thoughts, emotions, and sensations. Again, you are not your emotions! You are the creator and observer of your emotions. Emotions are energy. All you are feeling is pockets of intensely charged negative energy, linked to past wounds. You can choose to transform those sensations into positive energy, cultivating your true self in the process. You can make this choice right now. You can choose to relinquish your emotions and realize your real self.

Remember a time in the past when you handled negative emotions effectively. You've done it once, so now you can do it time and time again! Repeat this affirmation many times, and experience a shift in your emotional state and intensity.

Allow yourself to take relaxing deep breaths throughout your body in between each repetition. Feel the sense of calmness and love return to you, flowing through you. Do not rush. Rome wasn't built in a day! This may take time, sometimes a lot of it. The process may be very uncomfortable, but the result will be so worth it!!

Coaching and Positive Psychology

It's also important to emphasize that you don't have to deal with the process of recalibrating your thoughts and emotions on your own. Coaching sessions and cognitive behavioral therapy can play a role in bringing things to the surface. However, there are various approaches available depending on the needs of the individual; positive psychology can also be extremely effective. This field is based on the notion that focusing on strengths and weaknesses in human thoughts, feelings, and behavior is, as the name would suggest, more positive!

The researcher who can be best credited with founding this field is Martin Seligman. The former president of the American Psychological Association chose positive psychology as the theme for his presidency in 1998. In one influential paper, published during this year, Seligman wrote of "learned optimism," noting that:

> Psychological capital (PsyCap)—a recently developed, higher-order construct, applied to the world of work—has been hypothesized to aid employees cope with stressors in the workplace. [In this study], PsyCap buffered the impact of stress so that the relationship between stress and negative outcomes was reduced. In the case of Satisfaction with Life, PsyCap augmented a positive psychological outcome.[5]

Seligman believed and asserted that practices focusing on negative traits of our conduct could foster maladaptive behavior and negative thinking. Seligman was influenced by the work of Abraham Maslow, Rollo May, James Bugental, and Carl Rogers, which tends to focus on happiness, well-being, and positivity, as opposed to the treatment of conditions diagnosed through therapy.

Assertions made by positive psychology coincide neatly with the work of Napoleon Hill, who suggested that "any idea, plan, or purpose may be placed in the mind through repetition of thought."[6] Thus, by cultivating positive thoughts, we train our minds to follow a plan or purpose that serves our best interests. Equally, if we do the opposite and engage in negative thoughts patterns, we are setting ourselves up for the trap we have discussed extensively in this book: following a path through life that is limiting, inauthentic, and ultimately makes us unhappy.

Other modern work has built on these concepts. Psychologist Mihaly Csikszentmihalyi's investigations of what he refers to as "optimal experience" indicate that pleasurable experiences emanate from a state of consciousness he calls *"flow."* Csikszentmihalyi named his seminal 2008 work, *Flow: The Psychology of Optimal Experience,* after this concept, and noted that when people enter this psychological state, they experience deep enjoyment, creativity, and a total involvement with life— exactly the traits and life experiences that most people wish to foster.

Csikszentmihalyi demonstrates that by consciously ordering the information that enters our consciousness, we not only create an elevated state of mind but also unlock our true potential and experience a greatly elevated quality of life. In his work, Csikszentmihalyi outlines eight characteristics of this quality of flow, namely:

1. Complete concentration on the task.
2. Clarity of goals and reward in mind and immediate feedback.
3. Transformation of time (speeding up/slowing down).
4. The experience is intrinsically rewarding.
5. Effortlessness and ease.

6. There is a balance between challenge and skills.
7. Actions and awareness are merged, losing self-conscious rumination.
8. There is a feeling of control over the task.[7]

My Titanic Hit the Iceberg—Now What?

So, cultivating thoughts and feelings is extremely important. Equally, you cannot push back against them and repress negative sentiments. They have to be allowed to seep into your consciousness and then dissipate.

You need to allow your beliefs, judgments, biases, and everything that may prejudice your perspective on life into the space of awareness and conscious mind, so they can be processed and, effectively, eliminated. Perhaps we shouldn't even view emotions and thoughts as being negative per se, and instead should consider them to be restricting. Our beliefs and impulses restrict us—restrict our behavior, and restrict our potential—and it's only through the awareness and processing of these instincts that we can move to another level in our lives.

No matter what degree of trauma you have experienced or how restrictive your emotions have become, it is possible to work through and resolve any issues you have. Again, to mention the work of Dr. Gabor Maté, he has specialized in dealing with addiction and childhood trauma, people who have been to hell and back, and yet simply by bringing awareness of the foundation of their issues into their present, he has demonstrated that it's possible for people to overcome the most horrendous situations. You have to make that decision for yourself.

It's really a mindset based on your own attention and intention, alongside the active choice of thoughts. The motivational speaker and triathlete, David Goggins, includes in his ten rules for a successful life the key steps of reprogramming your mind, being present, controlling your thoughts, and visualizing the end result of your enterprise—all methods designed to limit restricting thoughts and create thought patterns related to growth and success.

Inevitably, you will find an approach that works best for you, whether this encompasses certain types of coaching, therapy, mindfulness, or other techniques. But you have to be aware and present with your situation first and address this before you can make significant progress. If you'd like to examine this subject further, please feel free to reach out to us, as we do specialize in this area.

Summary

In summary, often, in order to change your circumstances through your awareness, you have to change your thoughts around it, so your feelings associated with the situation change, as well. Once you have achieved this, your actions will change, your outcome will evolve, and your life will improve. While this is a linear approach to the subject, we would also advise more of an umbrella model, where several therapies and therapeutic remedies are combined, whether physical, behavioral, cognitive, or otherwise.

But the source and foundation of all behavioral and emotional problems are thoughts and feelings, so addressing the literal way we think and feel and then improving this is the only way to achieve ultimate success in life. Everyone who achieves any form of enduring success learns this lesson sooner or later.

References

1. Jia, X. Li, W. & Cao, L. (2019). "The Role of Metacognitive Components in Creative Thinking." *Frontiers in Psychology.*

2. Joyful Heart Foundation. (2014). *1in6 Thursday: The Emotional Pain Body, Part 1.*

3. Tajfel, H. (1974). "Social identity and intergroup behaviour." *Social Science Information/sur les sciences sociales,* Vol. 13, pp. 65–93.

4. BBC. (2021). "Emily Maitlis stalker 'will continue to brood and write letters."

5. Seligman, M. (1998). "Psychological Capital as a Buffer to Student Stress." *Psychology*, Vol.3 No.12A.

6. Hill, N. (1937). *Think and Grow Rich*, p. 47. The Ralston Society.

7. Oppland, M. (2021). "8 Ways To Create Flow According to Mihaly Csikszentmihalyi." *Positive Psychology.*

NOTES

_____

_____

_____

_____

_____

_____

_____

_____

_____

_____

_____

_____

_____

_____

Chapter 6

Weathering the Storm

HOWEVER HEALTHY our outlook might be, regardless of how well we come to know ourselves, and no matter how successfully we implement positive processes in our everyday existence, life will rarely go the way we want or imagine. It's easy to observe particularly successful people and assume that their lives have been an unerring, linear, upward curve of growth. That there have been no bumps in the road, no crises, no dips in performance, no disasters along the way.

Of course, that is a total delusion! Aside from death and taxes, the only certainty in life is that you will encounter massive problems and challenges. You will have difficult times when everything seems to be going wrong. And only through learning to effectively weather these inevitable storms you will ever experience any lasting happiness or success. So, this chapter will focus on an understanding of this issue, as well as some strategies and approaches to ensuring that you circumnavigate these tricky periods as efficiently and effectively as possible.

Firstly, it's important to reiterate that you must work through any negative thoughts and emotions associated with this process. You cannot repress, restrict, or reject these thoughts and emotions; you must address and process them. You must be mindful of the fact that if you do not satisfactorily resolve the restrictive thoughts and emotions you encounter, then you will never reach your full potential. And that is a huge part of weathering any storm that crosses your path.

There are several evolutionary mental traps that are waiting to ensnare us. It is vital we understand and avoid these, and instead instigate positive and constructive processes. In our model of the expansive self (awareness model), there are a few particularly significant forms of biases that can influence people during times of crisis, namely *impact bias, implicit bias, hedonic adaptation, and negativity bias*.

Impact Bias

Impact bias is the tendency people have to overestimate the length or intensity of future feeling states. This can operate on both a positive and negative level.

For example, we are sure many people can relate to the dread of going back to school after a holiday or returning to work after a vacation or any other such event in the future that we imagine will be horrible and uncomfortable! But then, we discover the reality of experiencing this event, after it has caused so much trepidation, is actually trivial. It's never as bad as it was in our minds!

Conversely, we can also internally build up the feeling of attaining cherished life goals into some state of nirvana and halcyon bliss, but then feel a crushing sense of anticlimax when we actually achieve them. This then feeds into negative reflections on whether all of the hard work and commitment invested in the process were actually worthwhile, which can in turn lead to profound feelings of regret or, equally, drawing the erroneous conclusion that what we need to do is seek another goal, then directing all our energy toward this new Promised Land on the horizon.

A study by Wilson and Gilbert in 2005 discovered that there are two primary causes of impact bias: *focalism* and *sense-making*. I.e., we have a tendency to center on one goal at the expense of everything else in our lives, and we have an intrinsic need to rationalize what happens to us.[1] Yet neither of these approaches to life is rational. It's neither healthy nor productive to exclude all other aspects of our lives in the pursuit of a solitary goal; in equal measure, not everything that occurs in an infinite and random universe can be rationalized as being meaningful. Sometimes, shit just happens! The more we accept this, the more we can minimize and process the emotional impact of seemingly important incidents.

Being aware of impact bias makes it easier to navigate. This also applies to implicit bias, although in some ways it is harder to overcome. Implicit bias is subtler and more diverse in nature, while, unlike impact bias, it does confer some benefits.

Implicit Bias

The term "implicit bias" was first used by psychologists Mahzarin Banaji and Anthony Greenwald, in a paper that argued that social behavior is largely influenced by unconscious associations and judgments.[2] Thus, implicit bias refers to any process whereby we have intrinsic attitudes without our conscious knowledge. You can probably comprehend immediately that this is the foundation of all bigotry, most obviously racism.

Implicit bias occurs at least partly due to a phenomenon described in psychology as *schema*. This concept refers to a pattern of thought or behavior that organizes categories of information or a mental structure of preconceived ideas. Schemas are extremely useful, as they enable us to make often well-founded assumptions about the world around us, meaning we don't have to understand and rationalize every single situation and object we encounter.

For example, schema associated with a tennis ball and an egg tell us that the former will bounce, if we throw it on the floor, whereas the latter will not bounce quite as readily! Thus, we expect the ball and egg to behave in accordance with our schematic understanding of them. If we bounce a ball and it cracks like an egg, or if we throw an egg on the floor and it bounces like a ball, we will deem either phenomenon an extraordinary surprise!

Of course, that is an example of a particularly rudimentary form of schema. In that context, creating a framework of understanding using schema is not difficult. Problems arise, however, when we use schematic inferences in relation to social groups and roles, worldviews, archetypes, and other more complex aspects of life.

We have experienced implicit bias in the most trivial of social circumstances. Once, we accompanied a friend of South Asian decent with representative physical characteristics and skin tone. This person is an entrepreneur and a high achiever. We were picking up food at a popular local restaurant. The front desk person immediately asked this person, "Are you here for Uber pick up?"

We were flabbergasted! This well-dressed and nicely groomed person gently responded that no, he wasn't. Two weeks later, this happened again! Clearly, the servers at the restaurant implicitly associated certain physical characteristics and skin tone with "Uber pick-up" drivers. It was quite clear, after discussion with the manager of the restaurant (who was extremely apologetic for her staff's behavior), that their intentions were not malicious, but their "implicit bias" resulted in their actions and behavior. The servers have since received appropriate training and education and have addressed the situation.

So many of our thoughts and emotions are implicit. Literally, we are not conscious of them. Thus, implicit biases in our attitudes are commonplace, and, in fact, it is reasonable to assume that every single adult possesses implicit biases within their makeup. (Often, children have yet to form these biases, but they cannot be ruled out of this process, either.) This means we can form stereotypical or misguided impressions of a wide variety of situations and issues, without being aware of this or being conscious of from where this perspective emanated.

Consequently, implicit biases are often better predictors of our behavior and views than our conscious values. This means we may believe that we're being informed and directed by certain principles, when the reality is we're actually responding to internal biases, which can be completely misleading and baseless. This can manifest itself in a multitude of different ways, but the important thing to understand is that it's critical to work through any potential implicit biases by bringing our conscious emotions, core values, and thoughts to the fore, and by consistently practicing mindfulness to keep ourselves grounded in the present.

Hedonic Adaptation and Negativity Bias

Furthermore, hedonic adaptation refers to the notion that, after positive (or negative) events—and a subsequent increase in positive (or negative) feelings—people return to a relatively stable, baseline level of impact after a certain, but variable, time period.

This explains why we feel good after purchasing that first house or experiencing our first marriage, child, vacation, or when we finally achieve that grand goal after a sustained effort or investment of time; but then, we slowly return to our baseline level of happiness or unhappiness. We return to our visceral discontent. Conversely, after feeling grief due to a major loss, death, separation, or any negative event, while people may experience often intense negative emotions, they nonetheless slowly return to their baseline. Thus, the pursuit of the hedonic treadmill will never lead to lasting happiness or fulfillment. Our minds have evolved this way to keep up with changes in the environment, which enables swift adaptation.

Furthermore, our minds seek pleasure and wish to avoid pain at all costs. Our minds are always on high alert to find and avoid problems. Hence, we are quick to recognize anything negative. Negativity screams at us! Are you annoyed due to the slightest comments from your partner or spouse? Or comments made by a colleague? This is why! We often disregard, or fail to fully appreciate, how much our families do for us and how much our friends support us. We have to consciously learn to recognize, appreciate, and cultivate positivity, because positivity whispers and negativity screams!

These are essentially common evolutionary traps, aspects of our mind and thinking that have developed to enable us to navigate a hostile and complex world. But they don't always serve our well-being, causing us to cling to some hypothetical future or bygone past.

Intentional Living: Addressing the Biases

A potential remedy to our inbuilt biases and mental traps is living more intentionally. We've already discussed the importance of core values; being constantly aware of your personal values can play a major role in this. If you're living intentionally, even if you encounter major challenges, working through these will become considerably easier. You will intrinsically understand that you're on the right path, and consequently, bumps in the road will be less disruptive.

Intentional living can be simply defined as attempting to live in accordance with one's values and developing attention to what matters most to you. In this book, we are focusing on values associated with self-improvement, success, and happiness, but intentional living has also historically encompassed religious and political values, which may lead to success and happiness, if these qualities are indeed important to you. The most important aspect, though, is to be aware of your fundamental beliefs, improvise them as needed, and be prepared to invest effort in ensuring that your behavior and actions reflect them.

Intentional living acknowledges that life consists of choices and that all attitudes and decisions can be determined by our conscious choices, rather than being dictated by past events or external factors (culture, peer pressure, etc.; see limited-self model) that are imposed on us. Once we know who we are and what we want to do, why can't we do it? If we invest time and effort in what matters most to us, inevitably we will be happier. We will also navigate the challenging times in our lives with ease and grace.

Mindset is always key in all forms of success. You cannot achieve success with a mindset that is obstructive to your primary goals. This is the basis of intentional living: you are aligning your mindset with what you consider important. Another important aspect of your mindset that will help you to keep going when times get tough is the value of cultivating a growth mindset, as opposed to having a scarcity mindset.

Scarcity versus Abundance

These two ways of thinking are fairly self-explanatory, but they have a profound influence over the outcomes we experience. Those who hold a scarcity mindset believe that everything required for future progress is, as the name would suggest, scarce! It's particularly easy to fall into this trap when you're beginning an entrepreneurial journey. You don't have the experience or established clients yet, so everything you want to achieve seems remote and in short supply.

This mindset originates in the most primitive aspects of our thinking and brain activity: the drive for survival. Our most base instinct is to survive, and this instinct will continually trick us into believing that what we need in order to survive is scarce. This tendency can be seen in animals with less evolved brain structures, who will simply be forced to investigate any and every opportunity to eat food, even if they're not hungry. Their brains simply tell them, "You need to eat to survive. Go over there and eat right now!"

In reality, our world no longer operates that way, and a scarcity mindset only holds people back. Conversely, an abundance mindset sees only positive opportunities and chances for growth. Those with abundance mindsets are grateful, creative, enthusiastic, and cooperative. They see all of the possibilities that human ingenuity can create. They seek practical solutions. Even when happy, successful, and fulfilled, they believe that their lives can get better, that growth is always possible.

In short, with a scarcity mindset, everything is inexorably closing in, receding, diminishing, becoming smaller; while with an abundance mindset, everything is getting exponentially bigger. There is endless room for growth in business and in life.

These are entirely contrasting ways of looking at the world, and consequently, they also both have their own lexicon of language. This is an important point: simply by mindfully and intentionally thinking and speaking about events in a certain way, you can change your mindset, the way you view the world, and, almost inevitably, your outcomes. For example, instead of speaking about "costs," talk about "investments." Instead of thinking about "security," consider life to be an "opportunity." Don't encounter "problems"; benefit from "learning experiences."

Creating an abundance mindset means actively fostering qualities that help germinate this way of thinking. People with an abundance mindset don't limit themselves; they think big. They focus on what they have, rather than what they don't yet possess. They're genuinely happy for the success of others. They have open minds that are willing to learn, and they never consider themselves to be experts in anything; there is always room for growth. All of these qualities are essential for success and vitally important when weathering the many inevitable storms that life will bombard you with.

Abundance Practices

And there are active ways you can develop this productive way of thinking and being. First, you can recognize and accept your weaknesses, while nurturing your strengths. Both of these practices enable you to enhance your self-knowledge, meaning you're less likely to feel threatened by other people's success or trying circumstances.

Visualizing your potential can also be highly effective. Harvard psychiatrist Srinivasan Pillay has conducted extensive work on the value of visualization, finding that visualization and action are intimately connected; visualization stimulates the same brain receptors as when you actually perform a task.[3] Essentially, this is a procedure that fools the brain into believing you've achieved a goal before you actually do it. Ask yourself what is possible in any given scenario and visualize the best conceivable outcomes. Then, you're actually one step closer to achieving them.

And jettisoning destructive and limiting habits to which you've become conjoined over the years is also particularly valuable. Negative thought patterns can become habitual, particularly if they were instilled in you at a tender age. Recognizing these beliefs, rooting them out by surrendering non-judgmentally to your cognitive awareness, rewiring yourself with positive affirmations, and repeating this process with regularity are all essential pillars of a strategy aimed at literally tweaking your brain chemistry and creating a new, more productive self. That's 4 Rs: recognizing, rooting, rewiring, repeating!

As you become more adept at developing this abundance mindset, you will find that so-called hard times not only become less frequent, but you don't even view them as hard. Everything becomes an opportunity, an experience, another chance for growth and knowledge accumulation. This mentality is hardwired in everyone who achieves success, and it is a keystone of personal happiness and fulfillment. If you focus on what you don't have, then you're promoting a scarcity mindset, and this will only delay your success and happiness.

Indeed, some people cling to this frame of mind like a cloak in a gale-force wind, and thus they never achieve the personal growth that would benefit them. They carry this scarcity mindset with them to the grave and, consequently, never taste life's sweetest fruits, achieving a mere minuscule fraction of their overall potential. So don't be that person!

Importance of Gratitude: Appreciating What You Have

One of the qualities that those with scarcity mindsets most obviously lack is gratitude. They're not grateful for what they have, and they're resentful because they don't have what they believe they should possess. And this is, more often than not, a comparative process. It's based on comparison with others. They want someone else's possessions or lifestyle or existence, so they focus on that, instead of cultivating their own growth.

This is why gratitude is such a key component in an overall practice of mindfulness. Research indicates that the most basic reflection on things for which you're thankful has a wealth of benefits, including more positive emotions, improved sleep, and even heightened empathy and kindness. Studies conducted by University of California Davis psychologist Robert Emmons found that regularly keeping a gratitude journal increased both well-being and life satisfaction.[4] This can be a document of the simplest and smallest things in life; it doesn't matter. We all have something for which we can be thankful, whether it's good health, personal relationships, or just some tasty food we consumed that day! Emphasizing these positives isn't an exercise in futility; it's an essential part of developing the mindset of a successful and happy person. The more you accentuate the positive, the more positives will enter your life.

The American writer and television producer, Rhonda Byrne (*The Magic, The Secret)*, has produced an entire series of books on the power of positive thinking, emotional well-being, and the benefits of developing a positive mindset. Byrne has become an evangelist for the power of gratitude journaling, writing that, "No matter who you are, no matter where you are, no matter what your circumstances or desires, if you make a gratitude list every day of the things you're grateful for, you will see your life take off! Gratitude is your magic wand! Whatever you point gratitude at increases, expands, and escalates, but you have to pick up that magic wand, and use it!"

It's also important to note that practicing gratitude is not confined to what appear to be purely positive events. Yes, you should feel grateful for the obviously productive experiences that furnish your existence, but the true practice of gratitude occurs when we are thankful for everything.

Author, thinker, and philosopher Napoleon Hill wrote, "I am thankful for the adversities that have crossed my pathway, for they taught me tolerance, sympathy, self-control, perseverance, and some other virtues I might never have known." Even in the face of disconcerting or inappropriate behavior, we can still respond with a sense of love and gratitude that will be far more beneficial than fighting fire with more fire.

Supporting Research for Significance of Gratitude

Aside from the research already mentioned, studies have repeatedly demonstrated that purposely cultivating gratitude can bring all manner of life benefits. Academic research has already demonstrated that gratitude can:

* Enhance your social standing: A study from the University of South Wales discovered that gratitude can help to improve personal relationships.[5] And further research published in *Educational and Child Psychology* found that keeping a gratitude diary enhanced children's sense of belonging.[6]

* Improve your physical health: There has been considerable demonstrative research in this area, but one particularly notable study, published in 2013, found that gratitude "correlated positively with self-reported physical health."[7]

* Improve your psychological health: "The Effect of Higher-Order Gratitude on Mental Well-Being: Beyond Personality and Unifactorial Gratitude," authored by Chih-Che Lin, indicated that "higher-order gratitude made a significant unique contribution to psychological well-being, self-esteem, and depression."[8]

* Reduce aggression and dissatisfaction: Cross-sectional, longitudinal experience sampling and experimental designs yielded converging evidence to show that gratitude is linked to lower aggression and higher empathy, in a 2012 study by DeWall, Lambert, Pond, Kashdan, and Fincham.[9]
* Increase mental resilience: Extensive research conducted by David DeSteno has found that gratitude improves mental resilience and is also connected to increasing our levels of self-control.

One final aspect of this that is well worth considering is gratitude meditation. This is a form of meditation that is particularly prominent in Buddhism, focused on expressing thanks for everything in your life. Again, studies have corroborated the benefits of this practice, documenting increases in feelings of well-being, decreased levels of depression, and improved empathy with strangers.

Again, this has been reflected in numerous studies. For example, Sirois and Wood found, in a study entitled "Gratitude uniquely predicts lower depression in chronic illness populations: A longitudinal study of inflammatory bowel disease and arthritis," that there was important support "for the relevance of gratitude for health-related clinical populations."[10]

Nezlek, Newman, and Thrash discovered that gratitude tends to promote higher levels of well-being.[11] And a randomized control experiment, conducted by Jackowska, Brown, Ronaldson, and Steptoe, found that gratitude "elicited increases in hedonic well-being, optimism, and sleep quality, along with decreases in diastolic blood pressure ... suggesting that subjective well-being may contribute toward lower morbidity and mortality through healthier biological function and restorative health behaviors."[12] In other words, simply by being grateful, you might live longer!

Forgiveness

When someone says or does something wrong, we frequently react negatively and carry a grudge. We seek revenge; we want to respond in kind! But we often fail to recognize that the only person we are hurting with these negative thoughts and emotions is ourselves.

This is, ultimately, counterintuitive, as forgiveness catapults happiness. Victor Frankl describes in his seminal work, *Man's Search for Meaning,* a psychotherapeutic method that involves identifying a purpose in life to feel positive about, and then immersively imagining that outcome.[13]

No matter what the circumstances are, no matter what wrong has been done to you, there is always a choice! You can choose to process your negative emotions and forgive. Forgiveness is now recognized as a powerful method to process accumulated emotional baggage and, in the process, to catapult yourself to happiness.

Above all, forgiveness is also about forgiving oneself and moving forward. Inculcating *unconditional love*—meaning approaching everything and everyone with love, regardless of the situation and circumstances—can catalyze forgiveness and compound personal growth, health, and well-being.

Law of Attraction

This chapter merely scratches the surface of the published research on gratitude and forgiveness, which has been proven to possess a broad palette of benefits. But attracting even more great things into your life is desirable, as well. This is where the Law of Attraction can make a big difference.

This is a philosophy that asserts that positive thoughts and emotions tend to bring positive results into a person's life, while negative sentiments tend to breed unfavorable outcomes. Having unwavering faith, clarity, and belief in what you want to achieve, regardless of current circumstances, is essential. Can you feel *now* the emotions you will feel, when you achieve what you want, regardless of what "is"? Can you trust, regardless of what is?

The fundamental point of the Law of Attraction is to develop the mindset that tends to result in happiness and success. This is not pseudoscience; it's something that can be observed in virtually every successful person you ever encounter. If you read an account of any top entrepreneur, almost without exception they will radiate positivity, often having maintained this sense of optimism, almost knowing things would get better during what appeared to be the most dismal circumstances on their path to success.

For example, Richard Branson slept on the concrete floor of a disused church when founding his record label, having left school with no qualifications. Everything that the system and society tells us about life would lead one to conclude that this was likely to lead absolutely nowhere! But Branson remained fully committed to his project, maintaining total belief in what he was doing. The rest of his extraordinary success is quite well documented!

If you allow self-defeating thoughts to occupy your cognitive space, then it would be churlish to expect positive outcomes to manifest. It's not beyond the realm of possibility, but almost without exception, those who allow negative sentiments to dominate their thinking will experience negative outcomes. Conversely, those who actively seek to be positive, to fill their lives with positivity, who create productive and optimistic thought patterns within their brains, tend to experience better outcomes in life. And, crucially, even when they do encounter the subject of this chapter—problems, challenges, difficulties, travails—they hold on to the belief that they will overcome them.

Furthermore, on an atomic level, we are all composed of energy, vibrating at different frequencies. The Law of Attraction, essentially the Law of Positivity, therefore asserts that by altering the frequency of our energy with positive thoughts, we will tend to manifest a more productive mindset, and this will then be reflected in more desirable results.

In his seminal work, *The Biology of Belief: Unleashing the Power of Consciousness*, the developmental biologist Bruce Lipton outlines the ways in which your mind and body interact and how your cells receive information. Lipton demonstrates that DNA is controlled by signals outside the cell, including the energetic messages emanating from our thoughts.[14] Referred to as *epigenetics*, this revolutionary understanding of the link between mind, matter, and the actual outcomes we experience in our lives has huge implications for the collective existence of the species.

Consequently, as your mentality shifts and you experience more success, you will believe that goals that once appeared to be impossible are suddenly reachable. You notice opportunities and open yourself up to new and exciting possibilities. This then feeds into your positive state of mind. You create a positive cycle, a virtuous circle of productivity, creativity, and activity. As David Schwartz, author of *The Magic of Thinking Big*, wrote, "Believe it can be done. When you believe something can be done, your mind will find the ways to do it. Believing a solution paves the way to solution."

As Joe Dispenza has noted, "Your body cannot differentiate between experiences that create emotion, and emotions that are fabricated by thought alone." What this means is that much of the anxiety, fear, stress, and other obstructive emotions you experience are created not by events in your life, but by thoughts in your head. Simply by changing the way you think, you essentially convince your body that everything is okay, transforming your energy from victimhood to being the creator of your own reality. You don't have to wait for it to happen; you can take control of how you feel, act, and even the outcomes you experience. A truly liberating feeling!

This is reflected in research on optimism, which has demonstrated that those who foster a mindset of growth, abundance, and positivity enjoy better health, greater happiness, and more success in life. This is precisely because of their mindset. They don't allow to fester the sort of negative and debilitating emotional states that can develop during challenging times. They employ a laser-focus on positivity, success, and all that is good and great about life. If you concentrate on creating desirable emotions and feelings, focused on abundance, gratitude, positivity, productivity, and joy, you not only create a mindset that enables you to push through the storms of existence, you also greatly improve your chances of creating more happy times.

In short, when you purposely change your self-talk, you transform the story of your life. As Eckhart Tolle has extensively documented in his work, true salvation is freedom from negativity.

References

1. Wilson, T. & Gilvert, D. (2005). "Affective Forecasting: Knowing What to Want." *Current Directions in Psychological Science,* Vol. 13, Issue 3, pp. 131-134.

2. Greenwald, A. & Banaji, M. (1995). "Implicit Social Cognition: Attitudes, Self-Esteem and Stereotypes." *Psychological Review,* Vol. 102, pp. 4-27.

3. Pillay, S. (2013). "Wired for Success: The Science of Possibility." *TED Talks.*

4. Emmons, R. & McCullough, M. (2003). "Counting Blessings Versus Burdens: An Experimental Investigation of Gratitude and Subjective Well-Being in Daily Life." *Journal of Personality and Social Psychology,* Vol. 84, Issue 2, pp. 377-389.

5. Williams, L. & Bartlett, M. (2014). "Warm Thanks: Gratitude Expression Facilitates Social Affiliation in New Relationships via Perceived Warmth." *Emotion.* Volume 15, pp. 1-5.

6. Diebel, T., Woodcock, C., Cooper, C. & Brignell, C. (2016). "Establishing the effectiveness of a gratitude diary intervention on children's sense of school belonging." *Educational and Child Psychology*, Volume 33, pp. 117-129.

7. Hill, P., Allemand, M. & Roberts, B. (2013). "Examining the Pathways between Gratitude and Self-Rated Physical Health across Adulthood." *Personality and Individual Differences*, Vol. 54, Issue 1, January 2013, pp. 92-96.

8. Lin, C. (2017). "The Effect of Higher-Order Gratitude on Mental Well-Being: Beyond Personality and Unifactoral Gratitude." *Current Psychology*, Vol. 36, Issue 1, pp. 127-135.

9. DeWall, C., Lambert, N., Pond, R., Kashdan, T. & Fincham, F. (2011). "A Grateful Heart is a Nonviolent Heart: Cross-Sectional, Experience Sampling, Longitudinal, and Experimental Evidence." *Social Psychological and Personality Science*, Vol. 3, Issue 2, pp. 232-240.

10. Sirois, F & Wood, A. (2017). "Gratitude uniquely predicts lower depression in chronic illness populations: A longitudinal study of inflammatory bowel disease and arthritis." *Health Psychology*, February, 2017, Vol. 36, Issue 2, pp. 122-132.

11. Nezlek, J., Newman, D. & Thrash, T. (2017). "A daily diary study of relationships between feelings of gratitude and well-being." *Journal of Positive Psychology*, Vol. 12, Issue 4, pp. 323-332.

12. Jackowska, M., Brown, J., Ronaldson, A. & Steptoe, A. (2015). "The impact of a brief gratitude intervention on subjective well-being, biology and sleep." *Journal of Health Psychology*, Vol. 21, Issue 10, pp. 2207-2217

13. Frankl, V. (1946). *Man's Search for Meaning*. Beacon Press.

14. Gustafson, C. (2017). "Bruce Lipton, PhD: The Jump from Cell Culture to Consciousness." *Integrative Medicine: A Clinician's Journal*, Vol. 16, Issue 6, pp. 44-50.

NOTES

PART III

OUTER EXCELLENCE

KETAN KULKARNI & FRANCIS YOO

Chapter 7

What is Authentic Success?

SUCCESS IS SOMETHING that virtually everyone wishes to experience in abundance. But it's important to remember something fundamental about it. Success is an abstract concept. It means different things to different people. The Oxford English Dictionary defines success as "the accomplishment of an aim or purpose." That is entirely logical, but it is the definition of this aim or purpose that is more important.

Juxtaposing Success

The situational aspect of success is critical. You can easily juxtapose two people who are reaching the end of their working lives, and the perception of whether or not they are successful can differ considerably.

For example, you might compare and contrast two men in their late sixties. One has had an extremely lucrative career in finance, has made tens of millions of dollars, has a massive house, owns expensive motor vehicles, boats, and an antique collection, and has all the trappings of a successful life.

Conversely, the other gentleman is much less well-off financially. He ran a small pet food company for many years and lived a considerably less glamorous and expensive existence. He lives in a small house with his family, owns a small hatchback car, has rudimentary possessions, and manages on a considerably less income.

Instantly, we would be attracted toward the first person as a symbol of success. But if you dig deeper beneath the surface, all is not necessarily as it seems. The guy in finance worked the sort of excessive working hours that we discussed earlier in the book. He drove himself to endure eighty-, ninety-, and even 100-hour work weeks throughout his life, in order to acquire the trappings of success on which he was fixated. This practice certainly rewarded him financially, but there were negative consequences as well.

His relationship with his children was distant, and he has two ex-wives. He has been warned by his doctor that his blood pressure is dangerously high, and he has also suffered from stomach ulcers caused by a drinking problem. The financier took to consuming alcohol with alarming regularity, using this as a tranquilizer to keep up with his extraordinarily demanding lifestyle.

As he approached the age of sixty-nine, this highly driven person reflected on the fact that he hadn't traveled, he hadn't seen the world, and he hadn't savored much of life and its myriad experiences. In fact, he hardly spent any time on his boat; all he did was pay the mooring costs! Now, past traditional retirement age, his body was failing him, his personal relationships had deteriorated, and he had more money than he could ever spend or use constructively.

By contrast, the second gentleman had cultivated excellent relationships with his nearest and dearest, involving them all in what had become a successful family business. It was never prodigiously profitable, but it always made enough money to bank some annual savings, which enabled them to take regular trips abroad and holidays, something the family always prioritized. All four family members traveled all over the world together, and once the children left home and moved on, the husband and wife continued this pattern as a couple.

While they only owned a modest home, its mortgage was paid off many years ago, which meant the gentleman could reduce the hours he invested in the business as he moved into his late forties. Effectively, he enjoyed semi-retirement for the last twenty years of his working life, just doing enough to keep things ticking on, while rewarding himself by exploring every nook and cranny of this beautiful planet. At age sixty-nine, the man's body is in perfect shape, he is still the same weight as when he was twenty, and he maintains an energetic and optimistic outlook on life, nourished by his personal relationships and believing he has enjoyed the richest fruits that the Earth has to offer.

Perception and Reality

Once all of this information has been presented to us, suddenly the notion of who is successful seems quite different.

The problem is that we too readily measure success by way of edifice. Superficial and external factors tend to define our definition of success, whereas if we assess the issue more deeply, then we might come to completely different conclusions. Is someone really successful if they have spent their whole lives in boardrooms? Maybe. But many people ultimately do not feel fulfilled by this existence and can never get back the time they have invested.

Currently, there is rampant evidence of job and life dissatisfaction, burnout, and unhappiness. There is constant pressure to achieve more. Life is extremely fast-paced with unclear and changing measures of success. Traditional career paths are rapidly becoming obsolete. Many working people often lack clarity and have a sense of going nowhere, despite hard and smart work.[1]

This is why self-awareness is intrinsically associated with success. It's virtually impossible to have success without self-awareness, as success can only exist on your terms. If it exists on the terms of someone else, then you can certainly say you have achieved the *dictionary* definition of success, but it may ultimately be meaningless to you, as an individual. What is the point in being successful if you don't consider yourself successful, or if you are ultimately unhappy with your life and life choices? Thus, there is a need for a comprehensive framework for success. There is a need for a clear definition, vision, and plan for success.

Let's consider another scenario. Let's imagine you are a twenty-six-year-old law student who has just graduated with straight As. Your whole life stretches out tantalizingly ahead of you. It seems like you have forever to both become successful and enjoy life, although people of a slightly older age will tell you this isn't the case! You're coming out of university with an excellent graduate degree, and you have already accrued a good stint of work experience. Even in a competitive job market, you will be a much sought-after candidate, so you have a wealth of opportunities and potential.

If you can put yourself in that situation, what advice would you give yourself? What would you prioritize? What do you believe is really important in life and will sustain your happiness and fulfillment? This is a completely blank-slate situation, and it offers you the opportunity to craft your life in an ideal fashion.

However, when we're actually in that position, we don't have the benefit of experience. We often don't know what we want from life, for the simple reason that we haven't developed self-knowledge and can often have a completely skewed impression of what is important. But it's a valuable exercise to consider yourself in this position and indeed to try to understand, at every stage of your life, what will benefit you.

False Comparison

Often, our instincts about life come from comparison. There has never been more information available about other people's lives at any time in human history, thanks to the prominence of social media. This phenomenon has had a multitude of unintended consequences, but one what has been cemented in particular is how we now live in a profoundly ingrained culture of comparison. Many people spend large parts of their lives looking at other people, comparing themselves to them, and often criticizing them, as well.

But in many cases, this criticism really arises as a tool to justify why the person making the criticism hasn't achieved something, which demonstrates the scarcity mindset. Or, if they're being abusive to someone whom they deem to be a subordinate, then the criticism comes from an insecurity about unachieved goals and ambitions.

In our view, this whole culture of comparison and criticism detracts massively from the growth mindset, because it distracts people from simply pursuing their own authentic goals. Why should you care about what someone else is doing? It doesn't impact you in the slightest. Success is always about success *on your own terms.* If you are attempting to live up to an image created by someone else—an image that is curated and therefore illegitimate in the first place—then you're definitely not following your own journey.

Yet this is an extremely common outcome for millions, especially young people, all over the world, who now have the monster of social media creating another nagging and nefarious influence in their lives. In our model of human development, this is a critical source of subconscious programming. The hours and hours people spend on social media translate into a critical source of programming, one that tends to instill this sense of comparison that can be debilitating to anyone's direction in life.

It's impossible to achieve success if you haven't adequately defined what represents success in the first place. And if this definition emanates just from external factors, how can it ever be appropriate for you? Seeking success is a quest for excellence, creativity, meaning, and purpose, and this has to come from within. That's why there is an almost intrinsic relationship between self-improvement, self-awareness, and success.

This is one of the important tools you require in order to achieve success. But there are other critical aspects, as well. The ultimate philosophy that drives your notion of authentic success is also really important. Discovering and understanding this can be a journey in itself. You can create a mindset profile, you can determine your personality type, and you can engage in other psychological and psychometric examinations. You can even go beyond this: you can study body language, spiritual subjects, etc. There are a wide range of models that have validity.

Aligning with Purpose

The problem for the generally accepted notion of success is that it is predicated on what someone wants to achieve, whereas the process of first identifying your purpose and meaning and then aligning your efforts in that direction is both an easier and more efficient solution. Only by identifying who you are and why you are that way can you hope also to understand what you need in order to feel successful.

And when we talk about the concept of success in this book, it is important to emphasize once again that this feeling aspect of the process is critically important. You can achieve a level of material and external career success that people will consider impressive. It can even be pleasant to receive the validation and approval of others. And some folk will even suggest that someone in a certain situation, perhaps someone who lives in a large house and has obvious trappings of wealth and traditional system-based success, cannot possibly complain about their lot. They have money, ergo they must be happy.

This is flawed reasoning. Nonetheless, it is easy to cling to a certain life situation and then consider it satisfactory. If you don't *strive* for the best and believe you *deserve* the best, how are you ever expected to *experience* the best? Still, it can be easy for a person with a net worth of millions of dollars who lives in a large house and has flashy cars or other attendant material possessions to believe that they don't have enough! We know many such people.

Again, this is a subconscious reflection of the social, political, and economic messages driven into our crania from an early age. We are told in no uncertain terms that you must achieve material success, that this is the epitome of happiness and productivity, and therefore many people find it hard to understand or even imagine how someone in those material and financial circumstances could feel unfulfilled.

Yet you know in your own heart whether or not you feel happy, successful, and fulfilled. If you do not feel this way, there is no amount of money, resources, material possessions, or even power that will tip the balance in a healthy direction. If you already have enough money to exist for the rest of your life, yet you feel dissatisfied, this indicates that the path you are taking through your life is an inauthentic one. This is undoubtedly bad news, but the good news is that it is never too late to change.

The reality is we all have competing needs (see Author Note at the end of the chapter). If we fail to acknowledge and service each of these needs, then we will lead an imbalanced life, and there will be no true success, no matter how successful we may appear. Because the true measure of success is internal not (just) external; if we don't feel successful, if we believe we've made erroneous choices, then our lives will never feel successful.

Success in Awareness

So, imagine the first scenario again. This time, the gentleman involved goes right through the awareness model. He establishes his core values, he develops a greater sense of self-awareness, and as a result, he fundamentally understands that his life needs to be in balance. He cannot neglect his relationships and then pick them up later. Productive habits need to be inculcated and instilled right now. He recognizes his business and financial needs but also his leisure needs, his downtime needs, his relationship needs, and also how these needs intersect and are of equal importance.

This was first documented and expressed in Maslow's Hierarchy of Needs, which delineates the various levels of requirements that exist in every human life.[2] This applies to everyone reading this book and its authors! Each level of Maslow's theory of human requirements also contains its own related needs, so it is only by addressing these that we will achieve the balance required for true fulfillment. Many driven people live without this balance, still believing they are pursuing their goals in a liberated fashion, but then, crucially, they experience no fulfillment when they achieve them.

Dr. Tal Ben-Shaar has become one of the primary communicators in the whole field of happiness. His book, *Happier*, analyzes why some people are happier than others, arguing that the concept of happiness is the most valuable currency you can acquire in this existence.

In particular, Ben-Shaar proposes that happiness is dependent on four quadrants related to present and future happiness. If you're willing to sacrifice your present moments for the desired future, then you are "rat racing." On the other side of the scale, if you are avoiding any and all discomfort and hard work, and instead indulging in immediate forms of entertainment, you are a "hedonist." The other two archetypes are, first, "nihilism," where you have lost your lust for life and lack both pleasure and purpose. The last is "happiness," where you are able to experience enjoyment in both the present and the future.[3]

Essentially, the balance here is between focusing on our goals and accomplishments while also enjoying the experience of the present and being able to relish this moment. Those in the rat rate erroneously believe, if they reach a certain destination, they will be happy. Yet this often disqualifies them from the possibility of enjoying what they're doing right now.

Conversely, hedonists fulfill only their present desires, giving no consideration to future circumstances. This leads to a lifestyle of immediate gratification, which can be fun for a while, but often hedonists fall to the earth with a jarring bump, when the consequences of their actions become apparent.

A Comprehensive Framework for Success

Instead, goals should be means not ends. As we have suggested previously, they should be aligned with your core values, with your calling in life. Ben-Shaar describes these as "self-concordant goals" and suggests that the key to happiness is ensuring we shift the expectations that we have of our goals, so they are part of the ongoing creation of our reality, rather than some point on the horizon to strive for. If we set goals that emanate from deep personal convictions, from personal meaning, then the whole process of working toward them becomes empowering, rather than an obstacle to be overcome.

A common myth that tends to be perpetuated is that people are driven by achievement, and thus we often believe we should seek goals that are obviously related to societally-recognizable achievements. True success is not just one goal or achievement. It needs to be sustained and long-lasting, rather than a tug of war between happiness and achievement. The reality of a successful and happy life is that it looks more like a kaleidoscope of various factors. So, you have a rich experience over a long period of time, rather than rely on plowing a lone furrow to bring fulfillment. Success is about achieving your own personal balance in the areas of happiness, achievement, legacy, and significance.

We will discuss happiness further in this book. But everyone recognizes happiness and joy as a feeling of pleasure or contentment in life. Achievement denotes accomplishments that measure favorably against others aiming for similar goals. Significance is a sense that you have positively impacted people you care about. Legacy is establishing a way to assist others in achieving success through your values and accomplishments.

Lasting success requires all these categories. However, without awareness, it isn't easy to do this. Highly successful people demonstrate considerable variability in setting goals for each category according to their personal values and desires. It's not just the amount of success in one category that matters; it is a proportionate mix in all four that determines lasting success. Success is also about a reasoned pursuit of enough, so being able to limit a particular activity for the sake of the whole.[4]

Fundamentally, this is why we have so many unhappy millionaires and billionaires: because their lives have been exemplified by a narrow focus on achievement. In fact, a limiting mindset is something that impacts even people who are hugely successful. Yet this can be very hard to identify.

For example, if you have a massive house and what appears to be a successful life, there is always the tendency to believe you should be happy with what you've achieved. Why would you wish to cause upheaval by massively changing your life, when you already have accrued a degree of security?

The answer is that it might make you happier! A new house, a new destination, a new country, and a new lifestyle may suit you far better than the one you have now. Taking the plunge can be scary and intimidating, but if it's what you desire in your heart, then it will always make you happier than sticking with a decent hand. Elements of our minds want security, routine, and certainty, so they trick us into being scared of the unknown. It's important to overcome this limiting mindset, as it will prevent you from achieving what you really want and are capable of doing.

Recognizing the Reverse Gap and Where you Came From

One useful exercise in this situation is to consider all of the things you've overcome in life, when you find yourself confronted with a difficult proposition. We are stronger than we think, yet we forget all of the challenges and obstacles we have managed to circumnavigate in our existence.

Every time we encounter a new problem, we tend to sink into an avoidance mentality. Yet this is completely unnecessary. Make a list of all the problems and challenges you have dealt with in your life, and you'll realize that you are much more formidable than you believe. You can achieve so much with the right mindset. The only barrier to achieving this is yourself.

Success is also, often wrongly, thought of as an individual pursuit. However, this is very wrong on so many levels. The people with whom you collaborate will be incredibly important to your success, but so are the personal relationships you craft and nurture. We mentioned the Harvard Study of Adult Development earlier in this book. This critical research has continually uncovered the fact that personal relationships are an important predictor of success and happiness in life.[5] No person is an island, so if you abandon and neglect your personal relationships, then you can expect any success to be fleeting, let alone any happiness and fulfillment.

And it's also important to consider the fact that success is constantly evolving. The concept of success differs from one person to another, to begin with, but it will also morph in form during your own life, as well. What you consider to be successful at twenty-five will not be the same as at forty-five, and the anatomy of success will change once more by the time you are sixty-five. So, when we talk about success in this book, it's important to understand that this concept isn't in stasis. It is changing continually all the way through your life, and you must evolve in order to remain on your authentic path.

This could operate in several different ways. We encountered one gentleman who initially worked for Nike as an IT engineer, but he recently moved into real estate investment. That's a big change in tack, but there's nothing to stop him from evolving further in the future. As mentioned previously, this can be something of an Achilles heel for people in professions, as they tend to remain static, locked in the same room for decades, and only breaking the pattern when they are offered retirement. This is particularly common in the medical profession and other highly specialized/skilled professions.

There is nothing necessarily wrong with that approach to life, and it does represent a relatively safe passage through this mortal coil. But we would argue that none of the people who achieved great things, or indeed great happiness, played it safe all the time. Life without risk is pointless. If you think about any of the people who have impressed or influenced you in your life, you can say almost unreservedly that they would have been risk-takers to some degree. You have to be willing to do that, to accept discomfort, if you want to produce something that really makes the world a better place, or even if you just wish to expand beyond the daily rat race.

This is nothing revolutionary or something of which most people aren't aware on some level. Most of us recognise that we need to do something to change our lives; we just put it off indefinitely. But you'll never achieve your potential if you keep delaying what's important. You must move the *Titanic* before it hits the iceberg. Once it hits the iceberg and suffers a total loss, it's often too late! It's always tempting to traverse the path of least resistance, but this will never ultimately sustain you. Anything worth achieving involves resistance and struggle. But the struggle is ultimately worth it!

Overwork or Workover!

You would think our whole concept of what constitutes work is something that should have evolved.

By the 1970s, automation had greatly reduced our requirement to work from a purely practical perspective. But by 2008, a Harvard Business School survey found that 94% of professionals were working more than fifty hours every week, with roughly half investing over sixty-five hours per week.[6] Instead of seeking a balanced life, the evidence suggests we are filling our days with inordinate amounts of work.

Hard work is undoubtedly an important component of success, but excessive work should never be considered a habit of a successful person. Healthcare researcher and physician Tom Fryers has identified three distinctive groups of people who work too hard:

1. Those who run their own business and feel that it can't succeed without them.
2. Those who are employed but wholly engrossed in their work and can't disconnect from it.
3. Those who work very long hours because it is expected of them by the culture, firm, or wider society.

And there are plenty of people for whom two or more of those characteristics apply. There are several warning signs of working too hard, and these include the following:

➢ You work longer hours than your colleagues.
➢ You can't "turn off" at the end of the day.
➢ You tie your personal worth solely to your work success.
➢ Your relationships are strained.
➢ Your work life is negatively impacting your health.
➢ You ignore hobbies and activities outside of work that used to bring you joy.
➢ You always feel behind no matter how much you do.

While we can self-select a life of hard work, and this can be fulfilling for some of us, we need to establish whether we have truly self-selected this lifestyle in full awareness of our needs. This is why being familiar with our core values is so important.

Hard work can be fulfilling and productive, but it can also cause psychological and physical problems, even death, if it continues indefinitely. For example, researchers at University College London found those who worked more than fifty-five hours per week had a 13% greater risk of a heart attack and were 33% more likely to suffer a stroke, compared with a control group of people working between thirty-five and forty hours per week.[7] And the Finnish Institute of Occupational Health found that people who worked long hours were 11% more likely to be heavy drinkers.[8]

Excessive working is linked with increased stress, burnout, declining mental health, relationship problems, loneliness, depression, and an increasing sense of dissatisfaction with life in general. This does not sound like the road to happiness!

Instead of working harder, the key is to work smarter. The foundation for this is the investment in self-knowledge and self-development that we discussed in the previous chapter. And then, investing some energy and commitment into exercises that promote both success and balance is hugely valuable.

★ Unplug from Technology

This is not about bashing technology. There is no doubt that technology has contributed hugely to our modern lives in a positive sense. But it is also responsible for making us accessible to a ridiculous degree! Consequently, the working days of many people continue as long as they are conscious! By being alive to notifications at all hours of the day, you are depriving yourself of critical rest, relaxation, and recuperation. So, make the effort to decouple yourself from all devices every day, and reap the rewards.

★ **Embrace Your Worst-Case Scenario**

Life isn't all about success, even for the most successful people. As British business magnate Richard Branson noted, "There will be lots of downs. Do your best to fight tooth and nail to survive. And if you don't survive, if you have worked damned hard, don't get down about it. There are a lot of successful entrepreneurs who have picked themselves up and started again." Fear of failure is often what drives us to work obsessively long hours, so when we relinquish the fear of failure, we go a long way to liberating ourselves from this irrational work ethic.

★ **Exercise and Meditate**

Healthy mind, healthy body—these are the two critical aspects of any healthy life. We have talked about meditation elsewhere in the book. Also, don't neglect your physical well-being—that would not be indicative of success or balance!

★ **Limit Time Wasting**

Identifying what is critical in your life is a productive process, but equally important is eliminating anything that gets in the way, or at least reducing it as much as possible. This might mean turning off email notifications, uninstalling that app or game you can't stop fiddling with, or even spending less time around people who gobble up your time or fill your life with negativity. Focus on the people and activities that reward you the most. Embrace efficiency.

* **Tweak Your Self-Talk**

As discussed before, positive and negative feedback loops are provoked by the way we speak to ourselves internally. There is nothing wrong with being demanding of yourself sometimes, but this needs to be balanced with compassion and praise. Similarly, training yourself to postpone short-term gratification when appropriate in favor of long-term gain is a crucial part of developing an abundance mindset.

You can also ask yourself key questions to raise awareness. What are you tolerating? What are you avoiding? What scares me? What do I dread doing? By getting answers to these questions, you raise your level of self-awareness and self-knowledge, while also providing yourself with an action list of items to address (see awareness model).

* **Journaling and Self-Reflection**

Another useful exercise is to write a brief journal of your day, every single day. This process allows you to reflect on what you have done and how you feel about it. This can help you build more constructive processes going forward. Furthermore, a Harvard study found that journaling employees performed significantly better than those who simply kept working until the end of their shift.

Journaling can be part of an ongoing process of self-evaluation and self-reflection, whereby you set yourself regular goals and targets, in order to replace bad habits with positive behavior. You can also seek feedback from others, as this can help to thicken the broth of self-awareness and make progress more rapid.

* **Creativity and Inspiration**

Finally, any working life needs to draw from imagination, so take some time every day to engage in some creative pursuits that inspire you. Schedule some time every day to do something creative. Read new and exciting books regularly, and listen to podcasts with valuable and engaging information. Don't just work endlessly. Keep your brain enlivened and open to new possibilities, and your life will be richer and your work better, as a consequence.

Summary

If you examine the life of anyone who has achieved great success, inevitably they will have faced massive challenges and even periods when it looked as if they had made terrible decisions.

Turbulence is normal, if you are chasing your dreams; you can't expect your rise to be an upward, linear curve. There are peaks and troughs for anyone in any field of excellence. What is important is to meet the challenges and have a longitudinal view of your life.

Successful people always have both eyes firmly trained on the long game; they realize that just because they have lost one battle, it doesn't mean they can't triumph in the war. This is the opposite mentality from most people in society, who instead seek for as many of their days as possible to be comfortable. They're happy to sit on the couch, watching television, because it's just easier than the alternative. Not that there's anything wrong with seeking some leisure time; quite the opposite. But if you want to achieve your true calling in life, then it is necessary to endure some discomfort and get used to it. You need to become comfortable with discomfort! It's important to get out of the patterns of behavior that are common among the vast majority of the population.

Equally, you won't achieve your proprietary version of success if your life isn't aligned with what is important to you and if you don't operate within a framework of self-awareness. If your life is an unending conveyor belt of constant work and striving, the chances are you will either crash or regret it in the longer-term.

Achieving success requires an excellent alignment of the qualities discussed here. It doesn't have to be perfect, but it can't be neglected, either. You need to understand what represents success for you. And then you need to take action in order to reach this point. The problem for most people in society is that they never come to understand themselves, they never recognise what a successful life would look like, and consequently they live an existence of inaction or obsession.

Which leads nowhere good.

Success is ultimately predicated entirely on mindset. Your inner work will provide the template for your external excellence. Achieving success on your terms requires that you take the model from the previous chapter, combine it with the lessons in this chapter, and continually apply and reapply it to your life. Only with internal focus will you ever achieve the external success you desire.

Further Work and Reading

We authors developed and now conduct an exclusive mastermind workshop to accurately identify, define, and map your personal authentic "success blueprint," so that you can craft your life by design.

Contact us at legendaryquestpro@gmail.com for more information.

References

1. Kulkarni et al. (2018). *Res Pract Thromb Haemost.*

2. Maslow, A. (1943). "A Theory of Human Motivation." *Psychological Review,* 50, pp. 370-396.

3. Ben-Shahar, T. (2007). *Happier: Learn the Secrets to Daily Joy and Lasting Fulfillment.* Actionable Books.

4. Nash, L. & Stevenson, H. (2004). "Success That Lasts." *Harvard Business Review.*

5. Mineo, L. (2007). "Good genes are nice, but joy is better." *The Harvard Gazette.*

6. Perlow, L. & Porter, J. (2009). "Making Time Off Predictable—and Required." *Harvard Business Review.*

7. Kivimäki, M., et al. (2015). "Long working hours and risk of coronary heart disease and stroke: a systematic review and meta-analysis of published and unpublished data for 603,838 individuals." *The Lancet,* Vol. 386, Issue 10005, pp. 1739-1746.

8. Virtanen, M. et al. (2015). "Long working hours and alcohol use: systematic review and meta-analysis of published studies and unpublished individual participant data." *British Medical Journal.* January, Vol. 13.

NOTES

Chapter 8

Leadership Myths Busted

AS WITH MANY of the words and terms discussed in this book, "leadership" is often a loaded concept. We all have a preconceived image of what leadership represents, and this is, to a great extent, promulgated by the prevailing media, culture, and society. Certainly, in the news media, people in positions of power and influence are often deemed strong and effective, if they are resolute to the point of being intransigent, never changing course or "flip-flopping," as it is often described. It seems our image of leadership is one of a workaholic who makes rapid and merciless decisions that are then followed through to their natural conclusion, regardless of any new evidence or evolving situation.

In fact, this entire image of leadership is one of the biggest cultural myths that continues to be perpetuated. A leader does not need to be an unquestioned and unquestionable authority, dispensing sweeping decisions derisively, while plowing through all obstacles in his or her path thanks to an overpowering and irresistible charisma. Not only is this not necessarily the best way to lead, but it also fails to pay heed to the reality that leaders are all among us. Leadership is not something that is bestowed on a person by their status or position. Rather, it is a mindset and cluster of behaviors that inform our everyday lives and the way we interact with the world.

By continually propagating this image of leadership, we overlook the fact that it is actually not something that can be defined quite so easily. Instead of thinking about leadership as being defined by status or attitudes, it is more apt to consider it in terms of outcomes. Leadership should appropriately be viewed as the ability to motivate, engage, and lead others to achieve a tangible goal or realize a vision; to guide others and play a role in their becoming the best versions of themselves. As soon as we define leadership this way, it seems certain that many readers will conclude that, for example, political leaders often fall considerably short of this ideal!

In this chapter, we will discuss aspects of leadership as they apply not only at a professional or vocational level, but also at a deeply personal level. We would like to bring your attention to how you can truly inculcate genuine leadership qualities and apply them to your own personal context and life, in order to realize your vision and promulgate personal growth. Developing good leadership qualities can accelerate your personal growth, enhance your joy and relationships, enrich your lived experience, and multiply your impact and legacy enormously.

Spectrum of Leadership

Leadership can be seen as a spectrum, something with immense scope. Rather than being something thrust upon us, leadership is something we can assume, regardless of our roles and responsibilities. Leaders do not need to be bosses or imbued with a particularly high level of authority or even responsibility. While the delegation of duties can be part of leadership, it is more accurate to view the role of leadership as being involved with engaging, motivating, and inspiring people, while also leading by example, exemplifying the values we wish to promote. Thus, the most successful leaders can communicate their vision in an inspiring way and generate enthusiasm among those around them.

True leaders become respected and recognized not by commanding and demanding, but by generating genuine trust and respect. The ultimate aim of any leader should not be about standing out from the crowd; instead, it should be to cultivate the best possible performance and mindset in every member of a team. We all have inherent and innate capabilities, strengths, and weaknesses that can either flourish and blossom or be neglected and wilt. Therefore, a successful leader will fertilize the particular qualities of the people with whom they work, enabling them to flower and experience their full potential.

This is another area where an abundance mindset is critically important. Leaders should never fear the people around them or believe that they are about to be deposed from their position, if they fail to retain an unceasing position of superiority. A leader needs to inculcate the ability to deal with obstacles and challenges, but a true leader is also able to concede when they do not possess knowledge, expertise, or experience in a particular area. Successful leadership means embracing the success of others and even reviewing the successes of opponents or rivals in a positive fashion.

Rather than being counterintuitive, this is instead indicative of an inner confidence, a belief that the appropriate mindset is in place and the correct course already plotted, in order to ensure success. We should celebrate the success of others, creating a positive mentality that enables us to better focus on achieving our own authentic version of success.

In accordance with this, there is no single compelling model that is the ideal for leadership. Leaders don't need to possess a certain personality type, nor should their skillsets be uniform and unchanging. While it is true that decisive, emphatic, and agile personalities are often perceived as qualities of popular leaders, research has demonstrated that people with a variety of personality types can be effective leaders. The ability to understand, comprehend and respond to the personality types of others is actually far more important than one's own character and preferences.

Emotional Awareness

Emotional awareness and expression are critically important, while nurturing two-way trust among teams and colleagues is also hugely valuable. If you can engender trust in other people, while also demonstrating that you trust them with important tasks, this will tend to promote a culture of inclusivity and integrity. In the process, it will ensure increased productivity and profitability. It should be emphasized, though, that agility is particularly important. The world today is diverse, which often results in complex working and interpersonal environments.

This goes against the grain of what has been assumed culturally and has fed into one of the most commonly expressed myths, namely that men are better leaders than women. Although this misconception has hopefully been supplanted in our culture to a great extent, the corrections has still not been reflected in positions of power and prominence. Yet academic literature and research point to the fact that men and women have equal capacity to shine as leaders across all fields.

It's also important to recognise that leadership is neither inherent nor innate. This is a critical aspect of the whole subject matter, as there is still a tendency to believe that not only are leaders born rather than made, but also that they do not need to engage in training and learning. Both of these assumptions are completely untrue! Leadership is undoubtedly a skill rather than a quality, something that needs to be honed rather than being based on biological determinism. It certainly shouldn't be denied that some people have inherent qualities that can lead to great leadership skills, but even they must not neglect their ongoing process of self-development and self-discovery.

Conversely, anyone can become a great leader and massively develop their leadership skills simply by instilling the ideal attitude, mindset, and practices. Becoming a leader in your own life means nurturing your skillset and training

KETAN KULKARNI & FRANCIS YOO

yourself to develop the qualities required to excel. This means that learning and refinement are essential tools in the armory of any successful leader. Workshops, courses, conferences, events, mentorship, coaching, and even just daily close listening to other people can all play a major role in the development of leadership qualities.

Active Listening

Many meetings, interactions, and communications are fraught with enormous challenges, such as disruptive behavior, indecision, and inadequate communication. These can ultimately disrupt relationships, leading to incorrect and ill-founded decisions, which then have the knock-on effect of significant delays in achieving desired outcomes. Active listening is therefore critically important. Yet this is not only a difficult skill to master, it is one that isn't always associated with leadership. We think of leaders as doers, not listeners. All this means is that our whole conception of what constitutes leadership is askew!

We cannot make sound decisions about our own lives, let alone decisions that impact on others, without first attentively absorbing all of the available relevant information. Failure to do this is failure to lead properly. In fact, we spend approximately seventy to eighty percent of the average day engaged in some form of communication, and about fifty-five percent of our time devoted to listening.[1]

So, if you want to lead in any area of life, mentors can actually be extremely important. This is something that many people in leadership positions overlook, as they believe that they need to be perceived as in control at all times. However, mentorship can play an active and continuous role in improving, and even discovering, personal qualities. You see much farther when you stand on the shoulders of giants, as the saying goes!

Leading Yourself

Above all else, leadership can be seen as a general process of self-growth, rather than being intrinsically associated with your job or position. In essence, learning leadership is an ongoing journey in which the destination is never truly reached. Personal growth is fundamental to becoming a leader in your own life.

Leadership isn't just about your job. Leadership can inform every area of your life, including academia, professional practice, entrepreneurial adventures, hobbies, passions, family time, and social activities. As we have discussed extensively, achieving true success requires successfully balancing all of the important aspects of life. This further underscores the importance and applicability of leadership principles in every area of your existence.

There is an overriding perception of what we believe to be a leader. It's someone in a suit, in a position of obvious power, with many people following them. But leadership should be viewed as being more about being a leader in your own life and taking responsibility. In an office environment, for example, you could voluntarily take on certain tasks that help things run more efficiently and that raise the morale of the workplace, as a result. These can be the simplest things, like keeping tea and coffee stocked up, arranging clubs and societies for socializing, or even changing printer paper regularly! Yet they can make real changes to the way that an environment operates, having nothing to do with titles, status, power, or even seeking recognition.

Historical Examples

There are many examples of people with these qualities sprinkled throughout history, often occupying completely different positions in society and working within extremely diverse fields. We wanted to pick a couple of potentially less obvious examples of leadership, to show how anyone can have a huge impact on their surroundings and even the wider world, regardless of their interests or position.

❖ **Albert Einstein**

Albert Einstein remains known all over the world for his mastery of physics and the incredible discoveries he made that paved the way for profound human progress. Einstein not only unlocked the keys to atomic power, but he also made crucial breakthroughs that led to such technology as GPS systems, televisions, digital cameras, the Internet, smartphones, and many other technologies.[2] Einstein's contribution to society can perhaps best be summed up by his own quotation: "Strive not to be a success, but rather to be of value."[3]

This mentality was reflected in the distaste the young Einstein had for the rigidity of academia. It seems that Einstein was never motivated by status and accolades; instead, he remained focused on practical achievements and progress. This principled position led the highly regarded scientist to take a variety of positions on social and political issues over the years, becoming an active leader of the international anti-war movement, while supporting conscientious objection. Einstein also made great efforts in his later years to encourage international cooperation in the new Atomic Era.

Einstein had many idiosyncratic qualities that contributed to his particular form of leadership. His appearance and dress certainly were not the stereotypical clean-cut with dark-suits one tends to associate with leaders. He also evolved from someone who had little regard for the field of mathematics into someone who recognized the importance and creativity of this field. Einstein was thus more than willing to occupy an unpopular position, but he was also prepared to concede when he was mistaken.

The particle physicist also strove to break through barriers created by conservatism, bureaucracy, and limited understanding of science. His passion for his field ensured that he was able to inspire others, creating an indelible impression on human understanding. This all emanated from his singular vision: Einstein's ability to perceive a better future for the human race. As he once said himself, "The leader is one who, out of the clutter, brings simplicity ... out of discord, harmony ... and out of difficulty, opportunity."[4]

❖ Bill Shankly

Another leader of note whom we would like to cite began life in the most modest circumstances. Bill Shankly was born in the small Scottish coal-mining village of Glenbuck,

Ayrshire. Times were hard throughout his upbringing, with hunger the norm for young people from his background. Shankly openly admitted that both he and his several brothers resorted to stealing vegetables from farms, biscuits and fruit from suppliers' wagons, and bags of coal from nearby pits. He said that he learned from this experience and vowed not only to work hard to secure a better future for himself, but also to be a better person.

Shankly worked in the local mine, when he left school in 1928, but he strived and dreamed of becoming a professional soccer player. Eventually, Shankly signed professional terms with Carlisle United and later made a major name for himself as a midfielder with Preston North End and the Scottish national team.

But it was as the manager of football teams that Shankly became a legendary figure, a successful leader, and a working-class philosopher. His mentality and outlook were always informed by this tough upbringing, which was reflected in one of his memorable early statements: "Pressure is working down the pit. Pressure is having no work at all. Pressure is trying to escape relegation on fifty shillings a week. Pressure is not the European Cup or the Championship or the Cup Final. That's the reward."[5]

Two *V* words were at the heart of Shankly's philosophy: vision and values. When he became manager of Liverpool, he outlined his intentions for the club and team. "My idea was to build Liverpool into a bastion of invincibility. Had Napoleon had that idea, he would have conquered the bloody world. I wanted Liverpool to be untouchable. My idea was to build

Liverpool up and up until eventually everyone would have to submit and give in."[6]

But in Shankly's view, this could only be achieved via a collective determination and commitment. And the collective extended beyond the team, the players, and the club, and into its fans and even the local community. Shankly spoke at a public event in the 1970s, where the people of Liverpool were congratulating Liverpool on winning a major trophy. He spoke to a crowd of thousands as people lined the streets of Liverpool, saying passionately, "I've drummed it into our players time and again that they are privileged to play for you. And if they didn't believe me then, they believe me now."[7]

Hard work and pride in your profession were also guiding principles for Shankly, and he constantly emphasized this when speaking about the game, his players, and his club.

"I think, if a man is playing in front of the public, who is being well paid, and he doesn't dedicate himself to the job, I'd be hard on him. If I could, I would put him in jail, out of the road, because he's a menace. My aim in life was, even in the Army during the war, you'd be given some horrible jobs. In the cookhouse, we had to dry about 6,000 dishes. And we cleaned the latrines. Well, if I had a job to do, even if it was scrubbing the floor, I wanted my floor to be cleaner than yours. If everybody thinks along these lines and does all of the small jobs to the best of their ability—that's honesty. And the world will be better, and football will be better."[8]

By the time of his retirement, Shankly had transformed Liverpool from an unfashionable and unsuccessful club to a highly successful powerhouse. He had created the "bastion of invincibility" that he'd said he would and had risen from the most derisory early life situation to be borderline worshiped by millions. And he achieved this due to a particularly proprietary vision of leadership that was focused on strong collective values, on doing the right thing for the greater good.

Summary

In short, leaders come in all shapes and sizes, occupying a variety of roles. And there are internal and external manifestations of their qualities. The important principle, when it comes to being the leader of your own life, is making a commitment both to self-development and to acquiring the skills and qualities that will enable you to make a meaningful difference in your life and the lives of others, in accordance with your core values.

Further Work and Reading

We authors developed and now conduct an exclusive mastermind workshop to accurately identify, define, and map your personal authentic "leadership blueprint" for your leadership development.

Contact us at legendaryquestpro@gmail.com for more information.

References

1. Lake, R. (2015). "Listening Statistics: 23 Facts You Need to Hear." *CreditDonkey.*

2. *Leaderonomics.* (2018). "Leadership Lessons from Albert Einstein."

3. *Brainyquote.* (2021). "Strive not to be a success - Albert Einstein."

4. *WildMind Meditation.* (2007). "Albert Einstein - Leadership Quote."

5. *The Scotsman.* (2013). "Scottish quote of the week: Bill Shankly."

6. *Liverpool Echo.* (2009). "Liverpool FC legend Bill Shankly - his most famous quotations."

7. The Shankly Hotel. (2018). "Commemorate the Anniversary of Shankly's Death."

8. *AZQuotes.* (2021). "Bill Shankly Quotes."

NOTES

_____

_____

_____

_____

_____

_____

_____

_____

_____

_____

_____

_____

_____

_____

_____

Chapter 9

Mastering Money

THERE CAN BE NO doubt that achieving success in life requires a modicum of financial success. That doesn't mean you need to become phenomenally wealthy. It just means that money is a necessity in this world. It's the key to living life on your own terms and simply cannot be neglected.

Means to an End

But it's important always to remember that money is a means to an end and not an end in itself. The ultimate goal of money is not to just acquire it; the aim always should be to acquire money so you can achieve your end goals.

If you have money, then you can make purchases you like and desire, but it also offers you many more choices. The most obvious example of the breadth of choices offered by money is that it can provide you with the means to stop or start working at your own will. That might not be everyone's choice, but it is an extremely difficult choice to make without some form of financial plan.

This idea is critically important in the context of this book, because many people completely lose sight of it. You would think it's easy to remember that money is a means to an end, but many seemingly successful people lose themselves in the unending pursuit of more wealth, believing they are becoming more successful as they accrue more. They believe that happiness will follow, if and when they acquire certain assets, things, and possessions or get somewhere in their lives. What they are truly after is how they will feel then they have those "things."

But the goal should never be to, say, accumulate $10 million. The goal should be to work out what $10 million will get you, to decide whether or not you need that, and then to scale appropriately. It's perfectly possible that you might be happy with a few hundred thousand dollars or need more than $10 million. Success is always relative, and above all else, it's specific to you. Don't pursue someone else's idea of success; pursue your own.

For example, we know people who have moved overseas and ended up living their ideal lifestyles without being anywhere near "rich" by Western standards. They've bought a property at an affordable rate, had savings leftover, and lived a nice life in an ideal climate. Sometimes, they've even started businesses, employing local people and paying them excellent salaries. The sky can be the limit, if you're willing to open your eyes and think outside of the box.

Money-Time Equation

Conversely, a lot of people spend their lives ensnared in the trap of never feeling that they have enough. They have the house, the swimming pool, the condo, the sports car, the 4x4, the Rolex, the yacht... and it's still not enough! They're still working their fingers to the bone for their high six-figure salary, skipping vacations, working eighty-hour weeks, and missing their family growing up. Then, one day, they get a stomachache. They just can't shift it. End up going to the doctors and are diagnosed with late-stage bowel cancer. Good luck taking your money with you!

That might sound harsh, but life is short and unpredictable. We never know what is around the corner. Some days, you roll a six, and other days, you can't catch a break. But this makes it all the more important to use your time wisely, as it's the only thing you can never get back. Money is vital, but it should always be viewed as part of a time equation. If you save money, then it can save you time later on, and this is the most valuable commodity known to the human race.

The work of Robert Kiyosaki is seminal in this regard. Kiyosaki highlights how employees and self-employed people often trade time for money. He suggests that, instead, we develop the mindset of businessmen and investors, who add value to make large sums of money and dismantle the equation of trading time for money. Thus, they gain superior control over their time and spend it according to their will and wishes.

This means we all need to assess, and often recalibrate, our relationship with money. We all have some form of relationship with money, as it almost inevitably provokes emotional reactions and often deep-rooted sensations.

One powerful manual on this topic is *Happy Money* by Ken Honda, in which he makes the following illuminating point. Everyone worries about money. Even if you're the richest guy or gal in the world, you will still think about money. It doesn't matter if you're rich or poor, you will still have an intrinsic attitude toward money, so it is therefore critical to understand and mend this relationship before it consumes you. Self-knowledge and self-awareness are always vital, and this definitely applies in the field of money.

The Right Attitude

It is therefore highly worthwhile to cultivate a positive attitude toward money. In relation to this, Honda suggests two particularly useful techniques. One relates to something we've discussed previously in this book: have gratitude.[1] Be grateful for the joys in your life and what you have now. Thank people who have helped you along the way, and be grateful to those who assist you in the future. Don't focus entirely on what you don't have; celebrate what you have already achieved.

Second, don't compare yourself with others. Compare yourself to who you were yesterday. This is such a powerful insight and yet something that virtually all of us fail to do, at least some of the time. The race isn't with other people. Remember: their goals could be completely different to yours, or they may be unconsciously staggering through life, like a beach ball bobbing around on the ocean.

Let us reiterate: some of the most seemingly successful people have zero self-awareness and often, therefore, experience zero happiness. Do you want to be like that? No? Then stop competing with them! Don't concern yourself with whether you have a billion dollars or ten million Instagram followers. Concern yourself with getting a bit better every day and working toward the goals that will sustain and fulfill you.[2]

The Psychology of Money

There are several ways to invest and well-known methods of planning for retirement. That's all great. That shouldn't be ignored. By all means, familiarize yourself with every aspect of financial planning, and set yourself achievable goals that will help you get where you want to be in life. But this chapter is more focused on the psychology of money, as this is at least as influential on our lives, and probably more so, than the pure mathematics of finance. How we see money, our attitudes to money, even our perspective on the wealthy can all inform our outlook and collectively shape the way we operate in life.

As with most important areas of life, many people buy into myths of money that color their views and perspectives. For example, it is not uncommon to hate the rich and famous. Isn't it ironic that most people want to be rich and famous, and yet they hate many rich and famous people to their guts? They constantly trash them, describe how the rich are unethical, are convinced they have amassed money by unfair means, and even describe them as bad people. How can you ever be someone you hate?

Equally, in modern culture, there is a prevailing attitude of placing the wealthy on a pedestal. Neither of these positions is particularly healthy. The important thing is to break down your personal attitudes and work out what they signify. Where did they come from? How did they develop? And how do they hold you back or influence your direction in life?

Healing Yourself

Until you're in awareness of your relationship with money, as with any issue, you cannot heal it and move forward. And "heal" is definitely the right word, as many people ultimately have an unhealthy and irrational relationship with this critical aspect of life.

Let's give you an example of this. We're all raised in different generations and eras, and even those people who lived through similar periods often have experienced vastly different circumstances. Different socio-economic conditions, different upbringings, different countries, and so on. So, it shouldn't be surprising that these circumstances underpin our attitudes toward money, saving, and investment. Studies have shown that people make investment or monetary decisions largely based on the experiences that occurred within their own generation, regardless of the prevailing climate.

This is, of course, poorly founded; decisions should obviously be made on the market conditions and options available at the time of investment or spending your money. But, generally speaking, we instead make emotional decisions predicated on our own underlying values and attitudes toward money. This can be counterproductive and even damaging, when our impressions of money have been formed in what is effectively a different world. That's why it's so important to become aware of our attitudes, our foibles, and our prejudices, when it comes to money and wealth.

For example, it's known that control—over your life, the people you mix with, and the activities you engage in—is the most important variable for achieving happiness. It is far more important than any status or economic indicator. The highest and most powerful expression of wealth is simply the ability to wake up and be able to say, "I can do whatever I want today." That applies whether you're a billionaire or even if you have little money, too.

Studies completely support this impression. For example, "Freedom and Happiness in Nations: A Research Synthesis" found that freedom is a key indicator of happiness, particularly for young people. And the researchers who worked on this paper also discovered that economic freedom is the most consistent factor in establishing a positive relationship with happiness.[3] This makes perfect sense: the more economic freedom you have, the fewer restrictions tend to be placed on your life. As Bill Hicks once said, "If you think you live in a free society, try having no money and see how free you are then."

Other studies have also corroborated this impression. "Happiness as an Expression of Freedom and Self-Determination" concluded that "the finding that happiness is related significantly to the degree of individual freedom is fully confirmed."[4]

And "Freedom and Happiness: A comparative study in 46 nations in the early 1990's" provided even more compelling evidence. This 2000 study, authored by Ruut Veenhoven, found that "freedom is positively related to happiness among rich nations." Interestingly, freedom was a considerably less important indicator of happiness in poorer nations, unless it was economic freedom. "A notable exception is economic freedom. Opportunity for free trade is positively related to happiness in poor nations ... Similarly, the relation between economic freedom and happiness is strongest in nations where capability to choose is lowest."[5]

Money, Freedom, and Myths

These conclusions shouldn't come as a surprise, but it is still interesting to see them confirmed. And it is important to emphasize the word *freedom*. Remember: money is a means to an end. If you have lots of money but no freedom (which would be a personal choice), extremely strong evidence suggests you will not be happy. Conversely, if you have relatively little money but loads of freedom, it is far more likely that you will be fulfilled.

Yet our relationship with wealth, material goods, possessions, status symbols, and other signifiers of money tend to be completely irrational. Much of this attitude can be attributed to modern marketing.

The story of the development of techniques related to advertising, marketing, and public relations was told memorably in the documentary film, *The Century of the Self*, which explains how society was shifted, intentionally, from a "needs to a desires culture."[6] This propensity is now ruthlessly exploited. We are told we will be happy if we have this car, this house, this product, or this lifestyle, even though we should know objectively that such promises are empty and completely lacking in substance or supporting evidence.

If we are ever to overcome this tendency to prioritize desires over needs, we need to live our lives on our own terms, rather than through some point of comparison. This priority, however, is perpetuated by social media, which helps to create a vast industry and culture of comparison.

In order to be happy, in order to be the best version of ourselves, in order to pursue our authentic goals and selves, we must sever the ties that bind us to an advertiser's image of what happiness should look like. There will always be someone wealthier, seemingly more successful, and attracting more attention than you. Forget about them. They don't matter, and they certainly don't matter in your journey. All that matters in your journey is being true to yourself and pursuing the goals that will make you happy on your terms. And all that ultimately matters for this is identifying what you need for your ideal life and then focusing on achieving this, rather than be sucked into an unending rat race that you can never win.

So, how do you get to where you need to be? Practicing gratitude definitely tends to promote a healthy mindset. The Arigato Principle from Japan, based around the simple concept of saying "thank you," can be valuable here. And the Law of Attraction is another important principle that can help to influence your outlook.

Visualization Techniques

Another useful technique, often used by competitors in sport, is to visualize what success looks like. This can seem like a tenuous notion to some, but actually its value has been well-established by scientific study. One influential study on brain activity in weightlifters found that similar patterns were activated when they lifted weights as when they visualized it.[7] In further research, groups of people who carried out virtual workouts in their heads were able to massively outperform a control group that just worked out.

There are many other similar studies, and research now indicates that thoughts produce the same mental instructions as actions. Cognitive processes in the brain are directly impacted by mental imagery, both positively and negatively.[8] By engaging in visualization, you are literally training the brain to be successful. Mental processes enhance motivation, confidence, self-esteem, and even motor performance. By training your brain to think a certain way, you can prime yourself for success and happiness!

The Napoleon Hill Money Blueprint

However, even with the best mental preparation in the world, you still need to take action, if you want to achieve success. It is here that a money blueprint, a documented approach to achieving financial success, is hugely beneficial. One of the most compelling examples of this is provided by Napoleon Hill, author of the international best-seller, *Think and Grow Rich*. Hill's blueprint to achieve wealth can be boiled down to a six-point process.

1. **Decide on a specific amount of money you need.** This might seem unnecessary; skeptics might wonder why you don't simply ask to be wealthy or for a lot more money. But studies by Edwin Locke suggest that those who set precise and challenging goals in their plans are more likely to succeed. There is, therefore, a specific reason underlying this specificity. Work out how much money you need. Set this as a goal.

2. **All goals require investment.** And the bigger the goal, the more investment is required. So, before you can set out on the road to achieving your goal, you have to accept that a certain degree of effort will be needed. This may mean that time and effort currently invested in other things will now need to be invested in making money and achieving independence. This could be your leisure time, moments with friends and family, or savings. Whatever it is, you will have to redirect and rebalance your efforts into achieving your initial goal.

3. **Set yourself a definite date** by which you intend to achieve your goal. If you choose a meaningful deadline, you

are far more likely to work toward it systematically, and far less likely to procrastinate. "A goal is a dream with a deadline."

4. Create a definite plan. Then, regardless of whether you feel ready to work toward it, **begin putting this plan into action immediately.** Rome wasn't built in a day, but the work to begin building Rome did begin in a day! The first step can be the hardest thing to do, particularly when you consider the enormity of the task ahead of you. That is why you need a plan and you need to put that plan into action every single day. Having an idea of what is necessary to reach your purpose will help you optimize your time and resources, making the attainment of your goal even easier.

5. Write out a clear and concise statement of the amount of money you intend to acquire and the time limits for its acquisition. State what you intend to give in return for the money, and describe clearly the plan through which you intend to accumulate it. Again, this might seem frivolous, but research indicates that people who write down their goals are fifty percent more likely to achieve them. Writing it down simply makes it seem more real.

6. Read your written statement aloud, twice daily. Once before retiring at night, and once after arising in the morning. He writes, "As you read, see and feel and believe yourself already in possession of the money." This is another affirmation and visualization technique, which has again been demonstrated to be highly effective. Kathryn J. Lively PhD wrote in *Psychology Today* that "affirmations are used to reprogram the subconscious mind, to encourage us to believe certain things about ourselves or about the world. They are also used to help us create the reality we want—often in terms of making (or attracting) wealth, love, beauty, and happiness." This plays a key role in the law of attraction, increasing your vibration and creating a higher level of energy that helps to attract the success and goals you desire.

Money and Spirituality

Now, this last point brings us to a key issue, one very important for us to discuss. Spirituality tends to have an uncomfortable relationship with making money, which can be viewed as selfish rather than enlightened. We're not here, the argument goes, to make enormous amounts of money. We're here to find inner fulfillment and joy.

That's an understandable position and perspective. But if you're seeking a fulfilling life in the modern context, it's inconceivable for you to achieve it without some accumulation of wealth. There is no compunction to be greedy. For example, there is a Tony Robbins video in which someone stands up in one of his seminars and states that he needs to acquire $1 billion to be happy. And Robbins steadily breaks this down and demonstrates how this is patently ludicrous! No one needs $1 billion!

However, you do need something. Of course, you can run away and live in the jungle remotely. That is perfectly feasible. We would suggest, however, if you've been raised in the West or any industrialized nation, this will be phenomenally challenging. But there can, nonetheless, be great joy associated with living a simpler life, connected with nature.

But if you want to live in the modern world, you cannot circumvent the need for money. This doesn't mean you need to be selfish. It also doesn't mean you can't give back to others. But there is no way around mastering money. We believe you can do this from a spiritual and ethical perspective. But you can't ignore it. Money is the elephant in the room when it comes to freedom, happiness, and success.

We are by no means uncritical supporters of capitalism, but it should equally be noted that the market system has played a role in producing and achieving some incredible things. We have more options, experiences, and potential available to us today precisely because of modern society, which has been predicated on a monetary system. We can never know how society would have developed without money, but we do know that many aspects of our lives are enriched by the products and services associated with industrialized society.

In our view, it is wise to embrace this and the freedom it affords, as long as it is done ethically and in accordance with your particular values. To be spiritual doesn't mean sitting in the gutter wearing rags with no material possessions. It surely means to explore your full potential in every aspect of human endeavors.

Mending your Mindset

Mindset has been a central focus of this chapter, and some exercises to help create the ideal mindset are certainly valuable. Many of our thoughts and beliefs about money are limiting. This needs to be addressed, as an abundance mindset is vitally important for achieving any form of success.

Getting to the core of your positive and negative thoughts about money is critical here, so simply writing down your thoughts about money, wealth, and successful people can be a useful exercise. Ultimately, you need to work through these obstacles in order to clear the way for your success. Did your parents or grandparents inform your views on money? Do you have a scarcity mindset? Do you feel resentment toward wealthy people? Or do you even have a habitual spending problem?

Once you have established these facts and excavated these issues, you will be ready to work through them. This can involve some real-world coaching. But we would also suggest, as we have in our model, that resolving restrictive thoughts and emotions around money of primarily importance. You need to reach a point where you can identify your personal needs, recognize that you have the right to acquire these and to be happy, and embrace the idea that everyone else's life path, achievements, and wealth should be meaningless to you. Other people can inspire you, but they are unrelated to your own life journey. The aim is to develop your mindset, so that you condition your mind to truly believe that you will acquire what you need to be happy and successful on your terms.

This book is not intended to focus on negativity. But the fact remains that there is a huge amount of negativity associated with money. Some of it is conscious; much of it is subconscious. It can come from our upbringing, from profound life experiences, or through external sources. Money makes the world go round, and so much of our discourse, debate, and dialectics are related to the dollar sign. It shapes our entire existence, not to mention our perception of the world around us.

Any entity that represents such a powerful presence in our lives can be exploited. It should therefore come as no surprise that the finance industry, marketing, advertising, corporations, and even governments and the state can take advantage of this. They prey on the discomfort people have around money, on the demons that cloud the judgment of so many.

Thus, we have to foster a mindset and relationship with money that is healthy, productive, and in full awareness of our requirements, if we are to be successful. The prevailing climate dictates this. Only when we have mastered our minds can we master money, and only when we've mastered money can we even hope to master our lives.

Further Work and Reading

We authors developed and now conduct an exclusive mastermind workshop to accurately identify, define, and map your personal authentic "money blueprint," so you can master your finances and financial destiny.

Contact us at legendaryquestpro@gmail.com for more information.

References

1. Honda, K. (2021). "Can Money Bring Gratitude, Happiness & Joy? Happy Money Expert Ken Honda Says Give It Away & See What Happens." *30Seconds.com.*

2. Rae, D. (2019). "10 Powerful Happy Money Lessons from the Zen Millionaire." *Forbes.*

3. Rahman, A. & Veenhoven, R. (2018). "Freedom and Happiness in Nations: A Research Synthesis." *Applied Research in Quality of Life,* Vol. 13, pp. 435–456.

4. Haller, M. & Hadler, M. (2004). "Happiness as an Expression of Freedom and Self-Determination." *Challenges for Quality of Life in the Contemporary World,* pp.207-231.

5. Veenhoven, R. (2000). "Freedom and happiness: A comparative study in forty-four nations in the early 1990s." *Culture and Subjective Well-being,* pp. 257–288, The MIT Press.

6. Häring, R. & Douglas, N. (2012). *Economists and the Powerful: Convenient Theories, Distorted Facts, Ample Rewards.* Anthem Press.

7. Hynes, J. & Turner, Z. (2020). *Positive Visualization and Its Effects on Strength Training.* Transylvania University.

8. Skottnik, L. & Linden, D. (2019). "Mental Imagery and Brain Regulation—New Links Between Psychotherapy and Neuroscience." *Front Psychiatry,* 2019; vol. 10, pp. 779-803.

NOTES

_____

_____

_____

_____

_____

_____

_____

_____

_____

_____

_____

_____

_____

_____

_____

PUTTING IT ALL TOGETHER

BEING THE CEO OF YOUR LIFE

&

HAPPINESS HYPOTHESIS

Chapter 10

The CEO of Your Life

DESIGNING YOUR IDEAL life means waking up your whole self. Taking full responsibility for your life, and accepting that you are fundamentally in charge of each and every aspect. We've outlined a clear pathway to achieve both inner and outer excellence, and when these aspects are aligned, then success becomes almost inevitable. There are many elements involved in creating this, which we have outlined throughout this book. Outside of the issues we've already discussed in depth, health and nutrition also play a positive role.

Ultimately, we believe that a happiness hypothesis is at the heart of all human fulfillment (see below). Essentially, we're looking for two quite simple things: the avoidance of pain and the experience of pleasure. If we have a life full of pleasure and devoid of pain, almost inevitably this will be happy and fulfilling. Within this model, spirituality is certainly a relevant pathway; i.e., seeking inner excellence as a method of salvation.

The Happiness Model

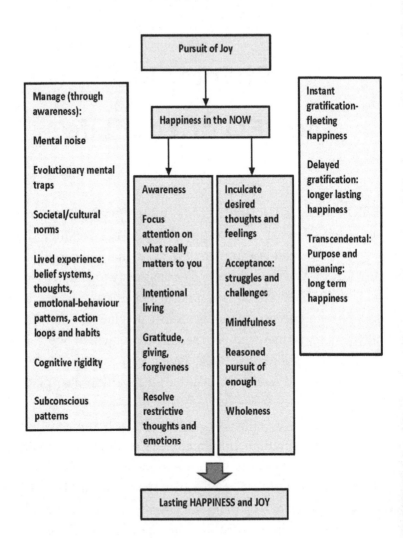

Externalizing versus Internalizing

When we talk about happiness and success, it is easy to externalize this whole process. The ultimate challenge and, if you like, battleground for happiness, though, is always inside. We so frequently account for the experiences of feelings but rarely consider the reality of just being.

This concept dates back to the earliest philosophers. Aristotle related the goodness of life to this inner excellence, as opposed to the fleeting pleasure that can arise from material enjoyment, including this concept in his guiding philosophy of *telos*, meaning the "concept of purpose."[1] This can be viewed as a contrast between instant gratification, which seeks to scratch an itch, and delayed gratification, where we seek to achieve something more substantial and constructive. It is the latter of these aspects of pleasure that is far more likely to lead to sustained happiness, particularly when we seek goals that add value and meaning to others.

As we mentioned in our models of happiness and success, when you're trapped in this state of the limited self, you fail to pursue the goals that will actually sustain you as a person. Awareness is so important to avoid this, whether it's being conscious of your core values, employing gratitude and forgiveness in your daily practices, engaging in mindfulness to raise your vibrational energy, managing your restrictive thoughts/emotions, or constantly having a mindset of expansion and abundance rather than that of cognitive rigidity and inflexibility. Being happy actually requires you to learn the process of how to be happy! It is not an externality; it begins within.

Mastering Awareness: A Philosophical Journey

That might seem daunting, as it requires a complete shift in perspective for many people. But, in reality, this realization is a profound gift, as no matter where you are in life, you can begin taking control of your awareness, attention, and cognition immediately, knowing that it is instantly moving you in the right direction. As you reprogram your subconscious, you will naturally begin to manifest not only the emotions that are desirable, but also the outcomes in your life.

This doesn't come overnight. Mastery of your mind and everyday patterns of behavior takes time. It requires consistent and conscious practice. This is where a technique such as creative visualization can be so valuable. This cognitive process involves creating a series of compelling mental images that are guided by your conscious thought. This in turn alters the emotions you associate with the subjects of the images. The more you practice this process, the more you are able to create the future you envisage. Creative visualization has even been used to create physiological changes, including the reduction of pain, while it is associated with a wealth of psychological benefits. And it can certainly be used to help create a spiritual pathway to excellence.

There are many different ingredients that combine to form a successful person. But one aspect of success is often overlooked. Virtually everyone who achieves success has some form of *philosophy of life*. They're driven, literally propelled forward, by this overarching perspective. And it also serves the purpose of underlining why they want to succeed in the first place. Throughout this book, we have continually made reference to the importance of your core values; these should ultimately underpin your own philosophy. Even successful people who haven't settled on their core values have, inadvertently, hit upon this critical aspect of fulfillment purely by developing a philosophy that is aligned with them!

Philosophy may seem like a grand word and one that many people wouldn't readily associate with their own existence. But all it really means is that you have synthesized a variety of information from diverse sources into a digestible form and use this insight to inform your direction in life.

That's exactly what we've tried to do in this book, to generate a roadmap that can be followed by anyone, regardless of their position and (perceived) status in life. Those things don't even matter. All that really matters is the direction you're going and whether it's rewarding for you personally.

Experimenting and Developing

Experimenting is part of the process. We like the concept of experimentation for taking control of your life because what you should be attempting to do is to design your life so it fits with who you are as a person.

That is really the core of this book and of human existence. Your life should embody your ideal concept of fulfillment, not that of someone else. The great writer and wit, Oscar Wilde, once said, "Most people are other people.

Their thoughts are someone else's opinions, their lives a mimicry, their passions a quotation."[2] This is surely even more true today than it was in the time of Wilde. Many people spend their lives attempting to live up to someone else's image of happiness and success. And it's neither productive nor necessary. You can choose your own path and you can continue to amend this path as you learn more about yourself.

The intention of this book is to help you begin the process of reorganizing and rediscovering yourself. And as we've passionately delved into this topic in our personal and professional lives, we'd be more than happy to field any queries you have about coaching or assistance.

Our outlook on life, as expressed in this book and other materials, is nothing new. It's something that has been understood for centuries, for generations, yet we somehow allow this wisdom to keep sliding away from our conscious experience. But the doctrinal religions, for example, have all expressed the notion that higher knowledge, higher purpose, and higher calling should be a critical component of our overall experience. Existential writers, such as Nietzsche, Kierkegaard, Krishnamurti, and even Dostoyevsky have written about the nature of existence and the meaning of life. And modern philosophers such as Eckhart Tolle, Gabor Mate, and Stanislav Grof have refined these concepts for the modern world, providing critical insight into the nature of reality, consciousness, and the self.

Traditional Philosophy

For Nietzsche, the meaning of life is to live authentically and powerfully, creating your own authentic goals and values. The German philosopher and cultural critic believed we are all individually responsible for what we do, who we are, and the world we live in.[3] His message was absolutely aligned with the notion that we must be the CEOs of our own lives.

Kierkegaard and Nietzsche have significantly different outlooks, yet the Danish theologian, philosopher, and social critic similarly asserted that any meaningful life should involve the diverse aspects converging to create a meaningful and coherent whole. There must be a meaningful goal at the heart of existence in order to be happy, and pursuing this goal should be the focus of existence.[4] Kierkegaard was, at heart, a Christian and had a somewhat evangelical message underpinning his worldview, but he still, rightly, acknowledged the notion of being guided by your core values.

Dostoyevsky was one of the history's most influential writers, and he frequently mused on both the nature of existence and the meaning of life. In *The Brothers Karamazov*, Dostoevsky wrote, "The mystery of human existence lies not in just staying alive, but in finding something to live for. Without a concrete idea of what he is living for, man would refuse to live, would rather exterminate himself than remain on this earth, even if bread were scattered all around him."[5] The Russian writer recognized that life must have purpose and meaning, and that identifying this is incumbent upon the individual.

Jiddu Krishnamurti was both a speaker and writer who has become an infamous figure in philosophy. Krishnamurti wrote, "Freedom comes with self-knowledge, when the mind goes above and beyond the hindrances it has created for itself through craving its own security. Freedom is at the beginning, it is not something to be gained at the end."[6]

This is a particularly interesting perspective, as much of our continual pursuit of monetary success at the expense of all else could seem to be attributed, at least partly, to this need for security. Krishnamurti suggested instead, as we do, that freedom and, with it, security can only come with self-knowledge.

Modern Philosophy

Eckhart Tolle is another totemic figure in modern philosophy. His outlook has always been focused on recognizing that this moment is the only thing that matters. This can be an obtuse concept for people to grasp at first, but it is simply centered on the notion that the purpose of life is to align yourself with what you are doing internally. Be present, and focus on the activity itself rather than what you wish to derive from it.[7] Your purpose is to divide yourself from the ego, identify your true self and purpose, and then make this the focus of your life.

Stanislav Grof, a Czech-born psychiatrist, has produced a mountain of work on transpersonal psychology and non-ordinary states of consciousness, with the aim of exploring, healing, and obtaining growth and insights into the human psyche. In *The Holotropic Mind: The Three Levels of Human*

Consciousness and How They Shape Our Lives, Grof wrote, "The message of so many spiritual teachers [is] that the only revolution that can work is the inner transformation of every human being ... Consciousness does not just passively reflect the objective material world; it plays an active role in creating reality itself."[8]

Success and fulfillment in the external world must begin with our own internal existence; until we have shaped this, we cannot hope even to know who we are, let alone create a happy life.

And Dr. Gabor Maté, an expert on addiction, simply suggests, "Our society denies us autonomy and meaning," and this ultimately leads to addiction in many cases.[9] While Maté is speaking primarily about drug addiction, this statement also has relevance to so many other examples of addictive and compulsive behavior, most notably workaholism!

When we have autonomy and meaning, we no longer need to strive for the pointless trinkets and status symbols that the media matrix deludes us into attributing with importance. Only our own meaning matters.

The CEO of Your Life

So, there are many, many examples of writers, thinkers, philosophers, and even scientists speaking about the importance of putting your authentic self at the center of your own existence. And once you begin to do this, your life will inevitably improve. However, there is no end to this infinite process. We would encourage people to continue developing in this direction, in order to refine and reform this evolution. Nothing is settled; we're all living our own scientific experiment on a daily basis, and this requires us to continually explore ourselves and what is meaningful in our lives.

That's what is meant by making yourself the CEO of your own life. *You* are the one in control. You're the one making the decisions. You decide the direction of your existence. You take responsibility for your success, your own happiness, your own life.

References

1. Hauskeller, M. (2005). "Telos: The Revival of an Aristotelian Concept in Present Day Ethics." *Inquiry* (Oslo). 2005 Feb; Vol. 48(1), pp. 62–75.

2. *Oxford Reference.* (2022). "Oscar Wilde 1854–1900, Irish dramatist and poet."

3. Martorano, J. (2019). *Nietzsche and the Meaning of Life.* TapInto.

4. Fernández, A. (2017). "Some Kierkegaardian Elements for a Philosophy of the Existential Subject." *Ensayos de Filosofía,* Número 5, 2017 (1), artículo 2.

5. The Human Front. (2020). *Dostoevsky on Purpose.*

6. *Neuropsych.* (2019). "10 Krishnamurti quotes on the meaning of life."

7. Andras, L. (2020). "Seven Quotes from Eckhart Tolle That Might Change Your Worldview." Medium.

8. *Inspiring Quotes.* (2022). "Stanislav Grof Quotes and Sayings."

9. *How to Academy Mindset.* (2021). Dr. Gabor Maté: "our society denies us autonomy and meaning..." and that leads to addiction.

NOTES

Epilogue

CONGRATULATIONS! If you have read all of the way to this page, you have demonstrated your commitment to redesigning your life. We have presented to you a step-by-step guide to inner and outer excellence that has been the product of many years of professional and personal investigation. We hope and trust you can apply the principles, concepts, exercises, and the philosophy of life presented in this book to your life immediately and consequently move the needle. Trust yourself and your journey and you will experience some amazing results.

We also hope this book has helped you awaken, or enhanced your existing awakening. It is possible that some concepts in this book did not resonate with you immediately. In that case, please allow some time for yourself to absorb them and reread the book in future.

Going through an evolution in your lifestyle and consciousness can be a challenging process, and achieving that paradigm shift in awareness is not necessarily an elementary proposition. It can take time. If you return to this book when you're further along the path to fulfillment and enlightenment—a goal we're all trying to reach!—you may find new wisdom, lessons, and practical takeaways that evaded you during your first reading.

We hope you keep this book where it's easily reachable and that you reread the concepts included, until they become second nature. We highly encourage all readers to complete all of the exercises, while also revisiting them periodically. Slowly but surely, you will reprogram your subconscious and consciousness, while bearing witness to a profound shift in the direction of your true desires.

While we present our perspectives and investigations around self-mastery, in no way is this book a complete guide to self-mastery. This is just the beginning. The only limit in this regard is the sky itself! The great masters in the world have demonstrated that there are many distinct pathways available, when you have committed to the journey of self-mastery. The spiritual pathway is among the most well-recognized, but the important thing is to pick the approach that meshes with your mindset and outlook.

Nonetheless, while spirituality may not be for everyone, ancient wisdom makes it abundantly clear that ultimately the aim of life is to find your true purpose and meaning and to surrender to the path of spiritual mastery, with the ultimate aim of achieving a superconscious state and oneness with the divine intelligence.

We are happy to connect with you further. Please reach out to us at www.thelegendaryquest.pro.

Thanks again for reading!

Acknowledgments

FRANCIS YOO:

I dedicate this book to Jeffrey Han.

I would like to acknowledge my friends and family who support, enrich, feed, and nourish me, especially my mother and father, particularly when I talk and walk the unconventional path.

I am thankful for the powerful influences on my entrepreneurial journey: my co-author, Ketan Kulkarni, Taylor Brana, DO, Mike Woo-Ming, MD, Maiysha Claiborne, MD, Mani Saint-Victor, MD, Peter Kim, MD , and the L&G Accelerator Crew, Sujin Lee, MD, Amelia Bueche, DO, Daniel VanArsdale, DO, Shawn Cannon, DO, Tara Lavery, Amir Baluch, MD, Christopher Loo, MD, PhD, Taylor Brana, DO, and Andrew Tisser, DO.

I am grateful for those who have helped me cultivate and develop Self and Wholeness: Lauren Davis, DO and Craig Wells, DO, Russ Hudson, Tao Semko, Daniel Atchison-Nevel, my Jungian psychoanalyst, Kathryn Staley, and my coach, Vikram Raya, MD.

For those whose work inspires and intrigues me: Tim Ferris, Seth Godin, Laura London, the Tofugu podcast crew, and Atlus, especially for their creation of the *Shin Megami Tensei: Persona* video game series, Capcom, especially for their creation of the *Gyakuten Saiban/Ace Attorn*ey video game series, and Gust/Banpresto, especially for their creation of the *Ar Tonelico/Surge Concerto* video game series.

KETAN KULKARNI:

This book could not have been written without the unconditional love, support, inspiration, and encouragement from my significantly better (p<0.0001) half, Saty. My children, Reeva, Risha, and Neil, make me experience and understand the fathomless equations of love, gratitude, and giving without expectations. My parents and grandparents nourished me in their loving environment, providing a rich experience by imparting invaluable life lessons and character building.

My close friends provide me with mentorship, guidance, encouragement, appreciation, and even reprimand me as needed. They are my infallible safety net. I am enormously indebted to my hundreds of teachers, coaches, and mentors, from kindergarten to the present day.... There are far too many to list them here, but all of them are/were amazing! Furthermore, my large friend circle further enriches my lived experience.

I want to extend a special thank you to my friend, colleague, and co-author, Francis Yoo, for his deep and whole presence and inspiration.

I am thankful to know about the great people who have or are walking the planet, including Albert Einstein,

Leonardo DaVinci, Nelson Mandela, Dalai Lama, Steve Jobs, Rembrandt van Rijn, Vincent van Gogh, Marie Curie, and many, many other world-class scientists, leaders, reformers, musicians, artists, writers, entertainers, celebrities, entrepreneurs, and thought leaders who have been, and remain, deeply inspiring.

In summary, I am the medium through which this book has been written. I realize I've always been standing on the shoulders of giants, and if I can see any farther than anyone else, that why! As I continue in my journey, I will remain grateful to everyone. I am beginning to realize that I'm a conscious being starting to experience and slowly understand the universal unmanifested source intelligence!

OUR INFLUENCERS:

We are extremely grateful to the following for their amazing work and contribution. This book draws many concepts from the work of these stalwarts (in no particular order):

Eckhart Tolle, Joe Dispenza, Simon Sinek, Seth Godin, Rhonda Byrne, Bruce Lipton, Kristin Neff, Martin Seligman, Morgan Housel, Robert Kiyosaki, Jonathan Haidt, Chris Voss, Daniel Pink, Jim Loehr, Tony Schwartz, James Flaherty, Ss Radhakrishnan, C. Radhakrishnan, Jack Hawley, A. H. Almaas, Martha Beck, Bob Burg, John David Mann, Mihaly Csikszentmihalyi, Mantak Chia, Don Miguel Ruiz, Hector Garcia, Francesc Miralles, Richard Bach, Ken Honda, Josh Kaufman, Ramit Sethi, James Hollis, Tim Ferris, Deepak Chopra, Richard Rohr, Paolo Coelho, Spencer Johnson, John Kotter, and many more.

For further information or communication contact:

Dr. Francis Yoo (SOUL Coach):
dr.francisyoo@gmail.com
www.DrFrancisYoo.com

Dr Ketan Kulkarni (SELF Coach)
ketanpkulkarni@gmail.com
www.savvyphysician.ca

Masterminds and Legendary Quest inquiries:
legendaryquestpro@gmail.com
www.thelegendaryquest.pro

About the Authors

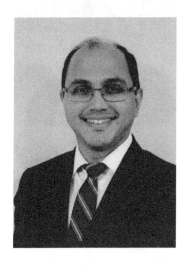

DR. KETAN KULKARNI is a physician, a clinician-researcher, a passionate entrepreneur, an advocate of financial literacy and independence through alternative income streams, an avid learner, a traveler, a photographer, an artist (and art enthusiast and antiques collector), and a music buff.

He is a certified LIFE coach with a focus on **SELF** (Success, Entrepreneurship, Leadership, and Finance) cultivation that draws upon his serial entrepreneurship, extensive leadership training, and executive leadership certification.

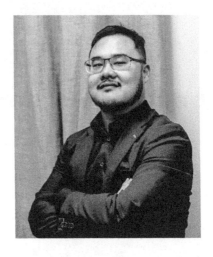

DR. FRANCIS YOO is an integrative Eastern-Western physician, guided meditation/cultivation practitioner, wellness and personal development consultant, an advocate for inner work, an electric guitarist, sushi enthusiast, and a video gamer.

He is a **SOUL** cultivation coach who draws upon a variety of experiences as a certified Myers-Briggs Type Indicator practitioner, Riso-Hudson certified Enneagram teacher, Glenn Morris's "Morris Modules," and KAP instructor.

NOTES

_____

_____

_____

_____

_____

_____

_____

_____

_____

_____

_____

_____

_____

_____

_____

_____

Made in United States
Orlando, FL
25 March 2023

31396309R00136